# Searching For Mama Coca:

## A TIME-TRAVELER'S GUIDE

By Bill Drake

And the community of writers

Who have searched for Mama Coca

Through the ages

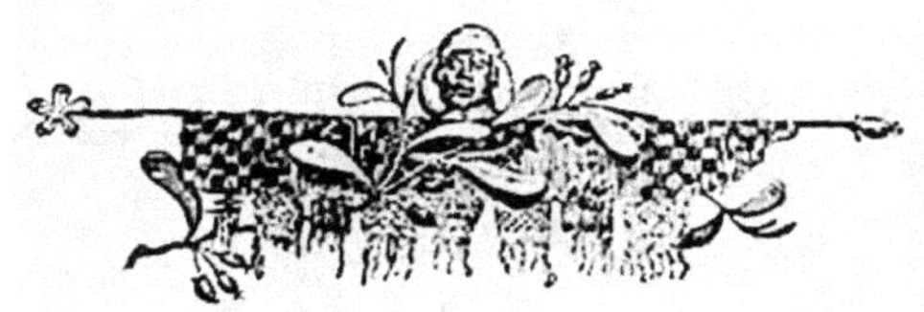

# Table of Contents

# Welcome Time Traveler

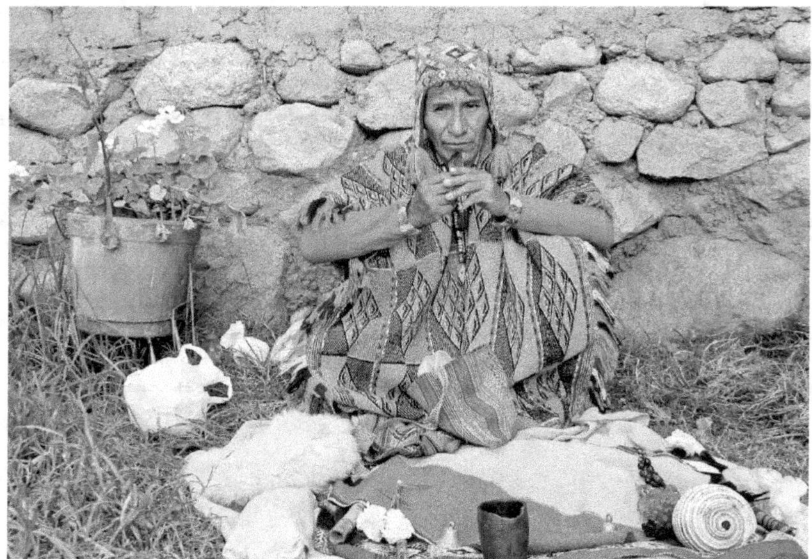

There is a strong and growing worldwide interest in the sacred medicine leaf of the Andes, and while I'm sure that there are many serious, innovative people growing and developing Coca Leaf medicines in many places, these experienced growers can't share their knowledge for unfortunately obvious reasons.

That's why I decided to reach into the distant past for knowledge that can be shared today, hoping to help along the liberation of Mama Coca and inviting growers to add their new knowledge to what I've gathered here from those who have gone before.

Throughout the book you'll encounter writers from hundreds of years ago, some with voices that strike an almost contemporary tone, as if they are communicating with us today. When they describe Coqueros of the Altiplano planting ripened Coca seeds, they are describing how Coca seeds are planted to this day in the high country of Bolivia and Peru.

I hope that you'll also enjoy hearing these writers talking as if they were walking a Cocal with a friend, sometimes arguing passionately about the best ways to age and dry their Coca leaf, prune their young plants, time their first harvest, and apply all their intimate knowledge of Mama Coca.

When a writer from 1880 discusses the best ways to extract Coca leaf using fine red wine, the fact that 170 years has passed since he wrote down his recipe is irrelevant to the delicious and healthful beverage and tonic he's describing. In fact, the 1880's *Vin Mariani* you'll encounter later in the book is being made again in France by Angelo Mariani's descendants, and a new chapter of Coca history is being written - Vin Mariani lives again.

In a real sense the voices in this book come alive today as they speak to us about every aspect of traditional and early European Coca cultivation and preparation as a natural medicine. But I hope you'll find that the real gem of this little book is the bibliography with convenient tinyurl links to dozens of forgotten Coca-specific books from the 16th through the 19th centuries. Many haven't been read in any detail for years, and some not for lifetimes. These books all now digitized and given life again in online library archives maintained by those blessed keepers of knowledge. I hope that the tinyurl links will make your access to centuries of long-lost Coca knowledge almost as easy as a quick digital click.

Because of the growing worldwide interest in the sacred medicine leaf of the Andes, I decided not to wait until legal public growing trials could begin. I'm sure that Coca Grows by serious, innovative people intended for developing Coca Leaf medicines and not for producing Cocaine are already happening in many places but people can't share their knowledge publicly yet. That's why I decided to reach into the distant past for knowledge that can be shared today, hoping to help along the liberation of Mama Coca and inviting growers to add their new knowledge to what I've gathered here from the sometimes very distant past.

Over a lifetime of study, I've come to believe that everything we need to know to grow and prepare natural medicinal Coca successfully and to create our own Coca Leaf medicines already exists in ancient books and journals. When we listen closely we are given far more than just "how-to" information through these still-living stories.

Mama Coca, as she once lived in the minds of people hundreds of years in the past, quite literally lives on today through their written words, and when we let them speak to us of their amazing insights and discoveries, they have wonderful things to tell.

Throughout this book you'll hear the voices of long-ago explorers and adventurers, scientists and zealots, botanists and naturalists, doctors seeking miracles and entrepreneurs seeking profits, along with assorted winemakers, philosophers, shamans, poets and rogues of every sort. Through their stories, musings and observations you'll gain diverse, personal perspectives into the long-disappeared worlds of the Coca Leaf medicines and Cocaine follies that grew from the European discovery of this sacred plant. The ancient Andean Coca cultures come alive again through the eyes of those who experienced, and in some cases dedicated their lives to understanding and appreciating that world, writing down their experiences and reaching out to future generations.

Not all the European interest in Coca was benign – not at all. For example, the Spanish discovered early on that the Inca rulers used Coca to work their Indian slaves harder, longer and with less food. They thought that was a pretty good idea and proceeded to conduct all kinds of horrific experiments in the name of increasing production of gold and silver for God and King, ironically working the Inca to death in the mines along with their former slaves.

Everyone who has written knowledgeably about it over the past three centuries tells us that growing excellent Coca Leaf is not difficult. According to this historical consensus, if you live in or can create the right environment, and if you have access to good seed or stock, which is obviously an issue in 2019, then growing Coca is not complicated.

The preparation of natural Coca Leaf tonics and medicines is also something anyone could do in a well-equipped modern kitchen, and the ancient Coca books you'll be linked to here are full of detailed Coca preparations, recipes, formulas, folk remedies and records of unusual experiments. In the 18th and 19th centuries Coca was sun-grown and greenhouse-grown worldwide from Paris to Bolivia to Java, and Coca Leaf medicines were treatments of choice for important diseases as well as in simple support of quality of life. The plain historical fact is that a cup or two of fresh Coca tea a day would revolutionize health in the 21st Century too, but that may take a while.

While there are many specific growing and cultivating, spelled out in as much detail as possible as you go through this book, that can make a big difference in the quality of Coca Leaf, and that will in turn affect the quality of medicines, tonics and teas made from the leaf, the Coca plant itself is almost universally considered to be a not very complicated or especially demanding cultivar. Well before electricity and certainly before lighting technology and high-tech indoor grows, traditional sun-growers and late the European and colonial glass-greenhouse growers managed to produce medical quality Coca Leaf just fine. My hope is that by reviving their long-lost knowledge and making it accessible I can help us all turn back in time to find to a healthier and more natural future.

# Section One: Lost Knowledge That Applies Today

## *Her Name Is Mama Coca*

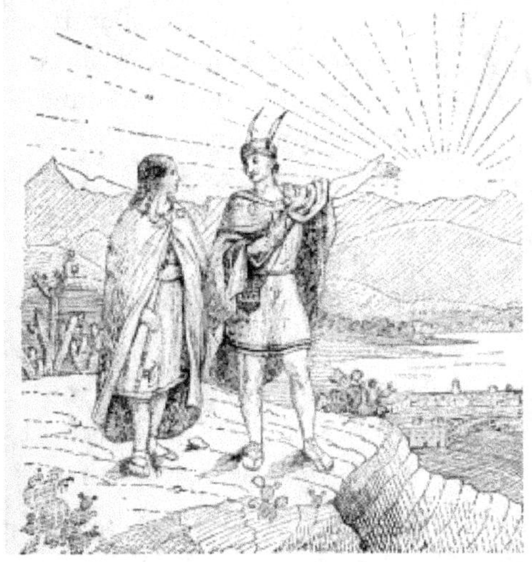

It would make sense that all the old journals and stories say that Mama Coca is relatively easy to grow. Mama Coca is certainly not as botanically complex a plant as Cannabis, and of course Coca carries her powers mainly in her leaf organ while Cannabis carries her powers in a biologically much more complex flower organ.

Leaf and flower organ comparisons aside, Coca and Cannabis share many of the same incredible healing powers and must also share the same generous Deva spirit. It's occurred to me that perhaps Coca is more like the Opium poppy in its basic simplicity, and in the relative simplicity of the chemical structure of its healing medicine, while Cannabis with its magical flowers and complex sets of healing medicines is biologically a very different being.

Mama Coca has been revered and celebrated by Andean people since the beginnings of their time on the planet for her benevolence and healing spirit. She blesses her children with good health, long life, creative energy, and physical vigor whatever their station in life.

Mama Coca is said to come to all who know her name and use the Coca leaf as it is intended to be used, but to reject and regret the Cocaine that the perverted chemists of Europe tore from her breast and inflicted on the world.

This Guide is dedicated to those who have come this way before us and have worked hard to pass on their knowledge. It's my privilege to be able to serve as part of that long line with this book of their collected wisdom on how to grow and nurture Mama Coca.

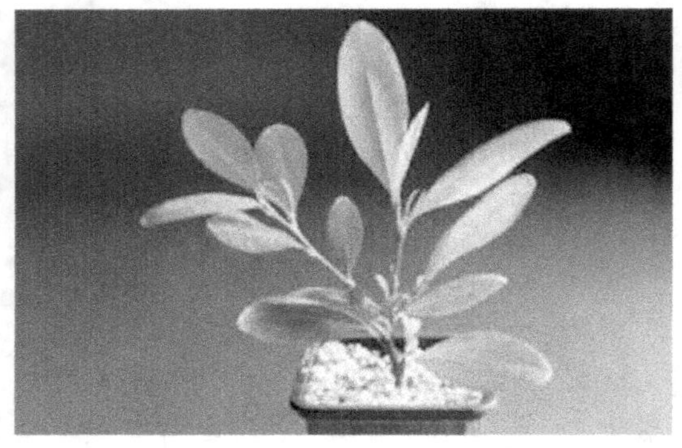

In this Guide you'll find detailed descriptions of producing Coca seed and taking Coca cuttings and then propagating, planting, cultivating, and harvesting them. This was all written in the centuries when planting and harvesting Coca for its medicinal leaf was normal and widely accepted.

Artists, singers, diplomats, bankers, police inspectors and others almost immediately began discovering not only the healthful but the delightful aspects of Coca quite early in the European experience. Many of them wrote about their experiences in charming and detailed fashion.

As I'm sure you already know, it is currently impossible to find a source of dependable quality Coca seeds or cuttings - unless of course you live in Peru, Bolivia or a few other countries and even then foreigners can't just buy Coca seeds or seedlings on the street corner, much less get them home safely. Neither Coca seeds nor Coca cuttings appear to ship or travel well without exceptional care, although there would certainly easy ways to deal with that if there were normal commerce in this natural medicine.

There are places in the world where it is still possible, according to travelers writing on the internet, to find escaped Coca plants from old 18th-19th Century plantations, some of which are described in the writings that follow, and in the now digitized original 1700-1900's sources you'll find cited with web links (when available) in the bibliography. Happy hunting if/when you get there!

As of this writing (2019) you can find people on the internet who offer Coca seeds, but there are no guarantees that they are legitimate, and there's a good possibility that they may be US narcotics police stings. I can't currently vouch for any suppliers. That sucks but it's real and the question is whether we let it stop us from politically asserting our right to grow for personal consumption or to share with friends any natural plant we choose, medicinal or not, recreational or not, bad for us or not.

However, until good sources of seeds and/or shippable cuttings develop, which I'm sure they will, and until people then start growing excellent medicinal Coca Leaf and putting detailed "how-to" videos on YouTube, which I'm very sure they will, I'm offering this little book full of links to past knowledge to help keep the spirit of Mama Coca alive while we're all working together to create that future.

## *Exploring Coca's Ancestral Home*

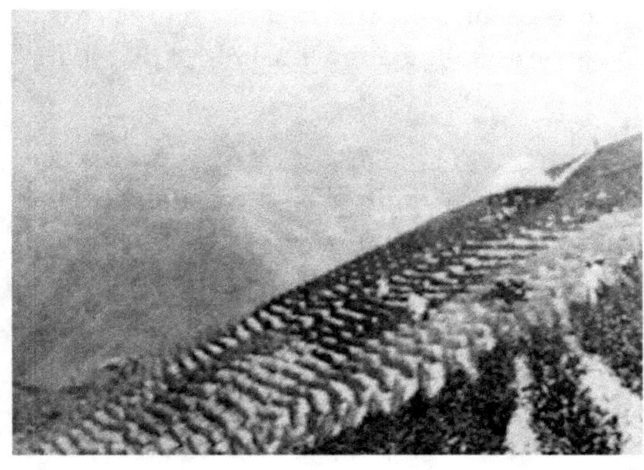

"On the descending slope of the Andes, from the bleak barren heights of the Sierra to the eastern Montaña, the soil at first thin gradually improves as the timberline is reached.

What at first appears like the scrawly brush of the barren mountain is soon found to be the scraggy tops of a more favorable growth beneath."

'The trees now loom into full view, weirdly draped with Spanish moss and bearing a host of parasitic growths in witness of the increasing humidity. As the declivity is now more steep, transition from the colder heights to commencing vegetation seems to be with an abruptness suggestive of a descent by balloon, rather than Nature's panorama of the shifting seasons here set on end instead of traversing the country."

"Everywhere there is a wealth of tropical plants, both wild and cultivated. The air is filled with the odor of sweet perfume from myriads of flowers, while here and there are sharply defined the clearings of the Cocals, or Coca plantations, which commence at an altitude of about 5,000 feet. The whole scene presents a marked contrast to the former bleakness."

"At times the mountains are surrounded by terraces, as though some giant stairway overgrown with an interlacing of tropical vegetation. In the utter barrenness of the western Cordillera terraces are built upon the bare rock with soil that must be brought from a long distance, but in the Montaña these are constructed for a different reason."

"The mountains are so precipitous that when a clearing is made the earth has no longer the support which it had from the roots of trees, and during a rain would be washed away unless held by the walls. These are built around the sides of the mountain, the height of the wall and the width of the terrace varying according to the inclination of the hill, while retaining an appropriate soil in which the Coca bushes are set out."

"Often these terrace beds are looked upon with envious eyes by some less industrious neighbor, and although the Indian is ordinarily honest and really too apathetic to be aroused to any serious transgression, the ease with which he may appropriate this desirable earth brought so ready to his uses may prove irresistible. The result is that the local tribunal has more occasion to settle the petty disputes arising from stealing a few bushels of dirt than for more serious offences."

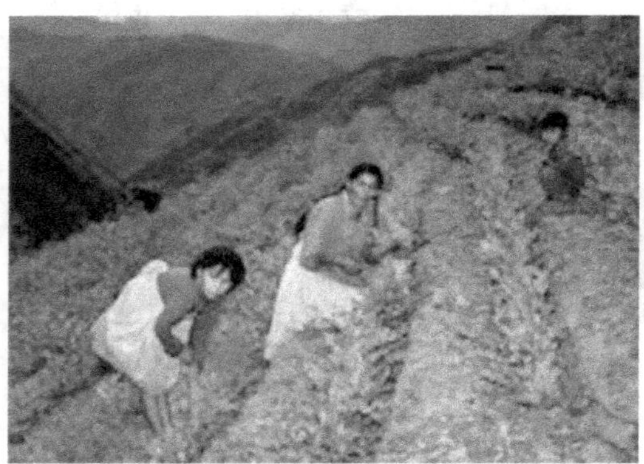

"The terraces - known as *Andeneria* - are usually built along the base of some hill where the declivity may afford aid to the Indian in making a clearing and yet where the drainage is suitable. On some slopes the inclination exceeds forty-five degrees, and the laborer is obliged to hold on with one hand while attending to cultivation with the other. There are many Coca plantations throughout Peru which are supposed to have existed for hundreds of years, and these choice locations are pointed to with reverential regard as having been continued from the days of the Incas."

"The raising of Coca is the chief industry of certain districts of the Montaña, and at one time the Peruvian government derived a considerable annual tax from it, but this is now only municipal, as at Huosa, where a tax of forty cents per quintal is imposed. In Bolivia the Coca traffic is said to be controlled by the State similar to the manner in which cinchona is regulated, the government reserving the right of purchase, a privilege commonly sold at auction to the highest bidder. In the mid-1800's the adventurer/writer Poeppig estimated the profit on a Coca plantation to be fully fifty per cent, and quite recently a prominent grower at Sandia said that a Cocal would pay all expenses in two years if three crops could be obtained, while often there are four harvests."

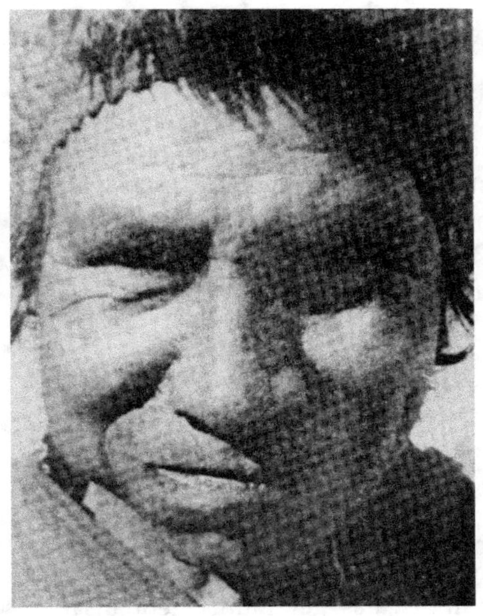

"Coca is still cultivated in accordance with traditions that have been handed down from pre-European civilizations, and there is still associated with it much of superstitious influence."

"Some Indians believe if a Coca bush be touched at its top by either man or beast the plant will surely die, while for a stranger to sleep near to a pile of drying leaves is considered dangerous."

"The Colombians say that no one should attempt to cultivate Coca who has not been favored with inherited talent in this direction, under the penalty of direful consequences, to say the least."

"Their women are not permitted to take any part in the several processes of the preparation of the leaf, which is similar to a restriction against women at a certain period in some of the French vineyards."

"Customs were so instilled in the laboring class of the Incas that the lapse of centuries has not changed them, and so the methods of cultivating Coca, described by Spanish writers immediately after the Conquest, may still be seen carried out with a minuteness of detail today. For just as Coca is indigenous to Peru, so too is the method of its cultivation, and each district has continued from generation to generation the traditions and processes of its predecessors, which, though varying in some trifle from those practiced in some other districts, are commonly similar throughout the Coca region."

"During the time of the Incas the terrace method of growth was that generally pursued, for east of the Andes the Montaña was thickly beset with unsubdued tribes of savages who resisted all attempts to infringe upon their territory. With the advent of the Spanish, and their recognition of the necessity for Coca in order to force the greatest endeavor from the Indian laborers in the mines, they pushed its cultivation further east and planted Cocals in clearings made for that purpose. As these were abandoned for other localities more convenient to their interests, the surrounding savages who had been driven from this land were quick to return, and so what at one time was a luxuriant Coca plantation soon became covered through neglect with the prolific growths of the jungle and reverted into an apparently virgin forest."

"So sudden may be the change here whenever cultivation is intermitted that it is difficult to appreciate its effect. The mighty trees of the forest are almost constantly falling, or are even pulled down by the parasitic vines with which they are encumbered, and once fallen they are immediately attacked and disintegrated by "a host of politic worms and insects, which crumble them into humus, while above and about these fallen hulks there is soon entwined the unkempt network of an impenetrable jungle. In some cases a tree may so fall as to span a stream and thus form a natural bridge, and such is the ordinary footpath over many a winding river."

"Man does not walk through the Montaña on the ground, unless paths have already been cut, but his way must be hewn with the machete, and then the walk is between an interlacing of vines and over the trunks of fallen trees, where progress at best is exceedingly slow and laborious."

"There is a wealth of everything, but it is of that wild, rugged and uncultivated nature which overpowers and even kills through a mere profusion. One may stand knee-deep in fuschias, geraniums, gentians and begonias, of a variety more choice than are commonly tenderly cultivated in more temperate climes, but which here are as great a nuisance as would be so many weeds where choicer growth is wished. Amidst an immensity of vegetation there are giant palms, tree-ferns, and an occasional cinchona towering far above one's head. Around are unnamed and innumerable dainty wax-like orchids, quite as common as is the hardy cactus of the bleak mountain heights, while butterflies, with the most gorgeous coloration, and of innumerable species, flutter like the fall of autumn leaves, but the beauty is lost in the annoyance of over-abundance."

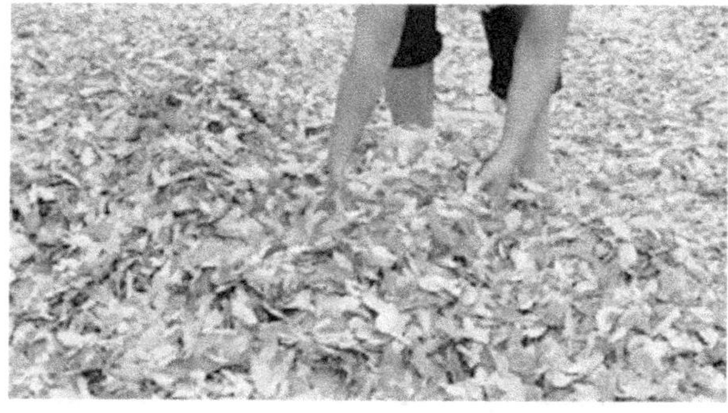

"The surface under cultivation in the little chacras, or Cocals where Coca is grown, is estimated by the cato. This is a piece of ground containing about nine hundred square meters or a little less than a quarter of an acre. Each Coca bush yields an average of four ounces of leaves, which dry out fully sixty per cent. Calculating the shrubs as set two by three feet apart, there would be upwards of seven thousand upon an acre of ground, or nearly eighteen hundred to a cato. A yield of four ounces from each bush would amount to four hundred and fifty pounds per cato at each harvest, and three harvests a year would yield an annual crop of thirteen hundred and fifty pounds of fresh leaves, or five hundred and forty pounds when cured and packed."

"Usually the Cocals are conducted by an Indian and his immediate family. When help is employed in harvesting the pickers are paid sixty cents of native money - at present equal to some twenty-nine cents of United States coin - for each thirty pounds of leaves picked. Adding to this an equal expense for cultivation, Coca under favorable conditions costs the planter less than three cents a pound at his Cocal. When the product is exported the expense of transportation by mule or llama over the mountains to the sea must be considered in addition."

## *Early Explorers Of The Coca-Growing Regions*

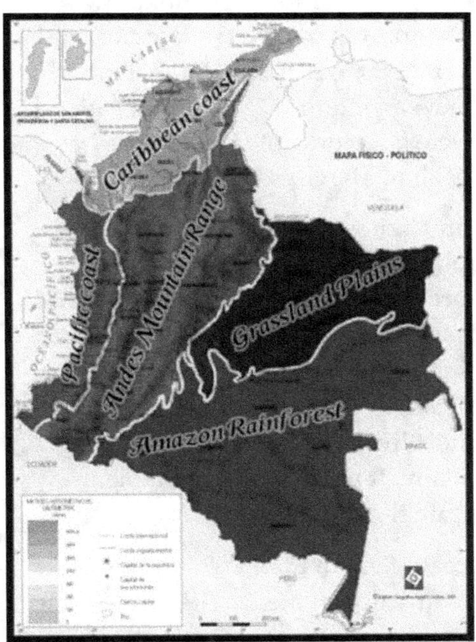


"Although the heart of the habitat of Coca is in the Peruvian Montaña from 7° S., north for some ten degrees, the shrubs are found scattered along the entire eastern curve of the Andes, from the Straits of Magellan to the borders of the Caribbean Sea, in the moist and warm slopes of the mountains, at an elevation from 1,500 to 5,000 and even 6,000 feet, being cultivated at a higher altitude through Bolivia than in Peru. "

"Throughout this extent there are to be seen large plantations and many smaller patches where Coca is raised in a small way by Indians who come three or four times a year to look after their crop. In some localities, through many miles, these Cocals cover the sides of the mountains for thousands of feet. During the Incan period the centre of this industry was about the royal city of Cuzco, and at present the provinces of Caravaya and of Sandia, east of Cuzco, are the site of the finest variety of Peruvian grown Coca."

"In this same region there grows coffee, cacao, cascarilla, potatoes, maize, the sugar cane, bananas, peaches, oranges, paltas, and a host of luscious fruits and many valuable dyes and woods."

"There are still important Coca regions about Cuzco, and at Paucartambo and in several Indian towns along the Ilnanuco valley, situated in the very heart of the northern Montaña and noted for its coffee plantations. At one time this region was accredited with supplying Coca for all Peru, which probably meant the mining centres of Huancavelica—formerly more prominent than at present—and Cerro de Pasco, where the mines are still extensively worked."

"Erythroxylon Coca appears to have come originally from Peru, and from there its cultivation was carried into Bolivia, Ecuador, New Grenada, and Brazil, in a word, throughout the entire torrid zone of South America."

"For some time, as a result of the extended consumption of Coca and for a still stronger reason, now that the day is at hand when the consumption of Coca will assume greater proportions, numerous plantations of Coca trees have been laid out in regions where that shrub was formerly unknown. We take pleasure in recording that these attempts have proved successful in the Antilles, thanks to the disinterested sacrifices of our friend, Dr. Bétancès. It is also with pleasure that we present anew an interesting communication made by the learned doctor to the "Société d'Acclimatation de France" as appeared in the Revue Diplomatique, 17th of March, 1888."

"Dr. Bétancès has succeeded in acclimatizing Coca in the Antilles. At considerable expense and after numerous shipments of seeds and the transportation of plants (this with the greatest difficulty) to Porto Rico and San Domingo, Dr. Bétancès had the pleasure of receiving a fine branch of Coca in full bloom, which was sent to him by Monseigneur Merello, Archbishop of San Domingo. This twig, which the members of the Society were enabled to examine, excited the most lively curiosity and won the commendation of M. Geoffroy Saint-Hilaire. It was raised from a plant which had been only eighteen months under cultivation."

"In Porto Rico the plant reaches a greater height than in Peru. It is therefore evident that the plant can be cultivated in the Antilles and that it may become a source of wealth to that country."

"Plantations like this would probably thrive in Corsica or Algeria, countries where the temperature at certain points is somewhat analogous to that of the tropics."

"It is a fact that this shrub does not attain its complete development except in countries where the mean temperature is from fifteen to eighteen degrees centigrade".

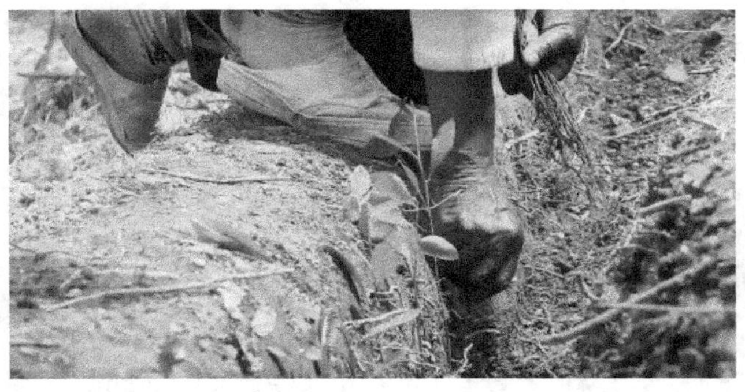

"But heat does not suffice; great humidity is also necessary to Coca Therefore it is met with principally on the sides of hills and at the bottom of wooded valleys which abound on both sides of the Cordillieras. Unfortunately, these regions are rather distant from the coast and they are, furthermore, devoid of easy means of communication; it is above all to this particular cause, the difficulty of transportation, that we must attribute the relatively high price of Coca leaves."

"The cultivation of Coca trees is begun by sowing the seed in beds called Almazigos. As soon as the plant appears it is protected from the heat of the sun by means of screens and matting; when it reaches a height of from 40 to 50 centimetres, it is transferred to furrows 18 centimetres in length by 7 in depth, care being taken that each plant is separated from its neighbor by a distance of a foot."

"During the first year, maize is sown in the interspaces, rapidly overreaching the shrub and taking the place of the screens and mats."

"The growth of the shrub is rather rapid, reaching its full height in about five years. But the time when it becomes productive precedes that at which it attains its complete height by about 3 years after being planted. After that, when the season has been especially damp, it yields as often as four times a year."

"Attempts have been made to acclimatize it in Europe, but so far without success. As early as 1869 the cultivation of it was tried in the Botanical Garden of Hyères, but no satisfactory result was obtained. We presented, in 1872, two samples to the appreciative and learned director of the *Garden of Acclimatization of Paris*, M. Geoffroy Saint-Hilaire, and notwithstanding all the care taken of the young plants, they failed to reach their full growth. Several frail Coca plants may be seen in the conservatories of the *Jardin des Plantes de Paris*, in the *Botanical Gardens of London*, of Brussels etc., likewise at several great horticulturists of *Gand*, notably *Van Houten's*."

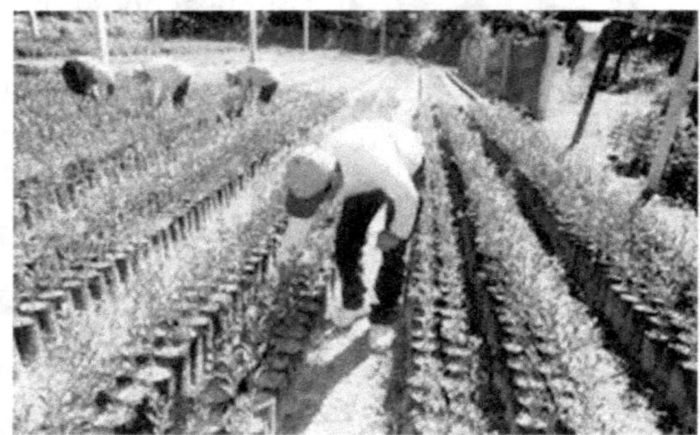

"There are fine Cocals at Mayro, on the Zuzu Piver, and at Pozuso—which are German colonies; at the latter place is located the laboratory of Kitz, one of the largest manufacturers of crude cocaine, whose product supplies some of the important German chemical houses. Still further to the northwest—in Colombia, there are a number of small plantations along the valley of Yupa, at the foot of the chain of mountains which separates the province of Santa Marta de Maracaibo, at the mouth of the Magdalena River."

"Eastward from the Montaña Coca is cultivated near many of the tributaries of the Amazon, and through some portions of Brazil, where it is known as ypadu. The Amazonian plant is not only modified in appearance, but the alkaloidal yield is inferior."

"Many early travelers and observers supposed they had found the original locality of wild Coca. Alcide d'Orbigny describes in his travels, having entered a valley covered with what he supposed to be the wild Coca shrub, but thinking he might be mistaken, he showed the plant to his mule driver, who was the proprietor of a Cocal in Yungas, and he pronounced it undoubtedly Coca and gathered a quantity of the leaves."

"It has been asserted that wild Coca may be found in the province of Cochero, and one of the former governors of Oran, in the province of Salta, on the northern borders of the Argentine Republic, claims to have found wild Coca of excellent quality in the forests of that district. Poeppig also described having found wild specimens, known by the natives as Mama Coca, in the Cerro San Cristobal, near the Huallaga, some miles below Huanueo. These examples closely resemble the shrubs of cultivated Coca collected by Martins in the neighborhood of Ega, Brazil, near the borders of the Amazon, and correspond to the wild specimens commonly found throughout Peru."

"In Colombia Humboldt, Bonpland and Kunth described Erythroxylon Hondense as the possible type of the originally cultivated Coca shrub, but there is a difference between the leaves of E. Coca and E. Hondense in the arrangement of their nervures, from which Pyrame de Candolle considers them as entirely distinct species. Andre speaks of Coca in the valley of the river Cauca as in abundance in both the wild and half-wild state, but an excellent authority denies that Coca is found wild in Colombia. The exact locality where Coca is indigenous in a wild state has, however, never been determined. "

"Though there are many Coca plants growing throughout the Montaña outside of cultivation, it is presumed that these are examples where the seeds of the plant have either been unintentionally scattered or else are the remains of some neglected plantation where might have flourished a vigorous Cocal under the Spanish reign. There are evidences of these scattered shrubs throughout the entire region where Coca will grow, but there is no historical data to base a conclusion that these represent wild plants of any distinct original variety, while the weight of testimony indicates that they are examples of the traditional plant which have escaped from cultivation."

## Section Two: Truxillo (Peruvian) & Huanuco (Bolivian) Coca Leaf

"The Coca which comes to the markets of the commercial world is broadly grouped in two varieties, the Bolivian or Huanuco and the Peruvian or Truxillo variety, the characteristic difference between the two varieties being that the Bolivian leaf is thick, dark green colored above and yellowish beneath, while the Peruvian leaf is smaller, more delicate, light color and grayish beneath. Manufacturers of cocaine use practically nothing except the Bolivian or Huanuco Coca, which contains the highest percentage of cocaine and the least quantity of associate alkaloids, which cocaine manufacturers have regarded as "objectionable" because they will not crystallize. While medicinally the Coca yielding a combination of alkaloids is preferred, the two varieties of leaf are entirely distinct as to flavor, being more pronouncedly bitter in proportion to the relative amount of cocaine present.

"Any attempt to describe Coca as a whole from any one variety, it will be seen, must be confusional, Bolivian Coca being rich in cocaine, while Peruvian Coca is richer in aromatic alkaloids. This variation is still maintained in the plants grown artificially at Paris and in the East.

"Plants and seeds of several varieties of Coca have been distributed to the botanical gardens of the English colonies at Demerara, Ceylon, Darjeeling, and Alipore, where they are cultivated in a commercial way and where they have been carefully studied under the new conditions of environment. Having in mind the history of cinchona, which had been taken from its native home in the Montaña of Peru and so successfully cultivated in the East, it seems a natural inference that Coca may also be grown scientifically under similar facilities where the possibility for distribution would be superior to the crude Andean methods. Certain parts of Java are particularly suggestive of the Coca region of Peru. The country is traversed by two chains of mountains which are volcanic, and, as in the Andean region, the vegetation varies with the altitude. From the seaboard to an elevation of 2,000 feet the growth is of a tropical nature, and rice, cotton and spices abound. Above this to 4,500 feet coffee, tea and sugar are raised, while still higher, to 7,500 feet, only the plants of a temperate region can be grown.

"There are many details essential in the cultivation of tea and coffee which suggest similar necessities in the cultivation of Coca. In Ceylon the best coffee is grown from 3,000 to 4,500 feet above the sea, where rain is frequent and the temperature moderate, and, like Coca, the higher the altitude in which the shrub can be cultivated without frost, the better is the quality of the product. Although the yield may be less, the aromatic principles are more abundant and finer than that produced in the lowlands. Similar hilly ground where there is good drainage is best adapted for the growth of tea. The shrubs do not yield leaves fit for picking before the third year, the produce increasing yearly until the tenth year. The yield from the tea plant is about the same as that from Coca, but the young leaves of tea are usually gathered, while only the matured leaves of Coca are picked.

"The climate, the environment, the method of cultivation and even the uses all seem paralleled in tea, coffee and Coca, but the benefits of application are immensely in favor of Coca.

### *Huanuco Coca Leaf*

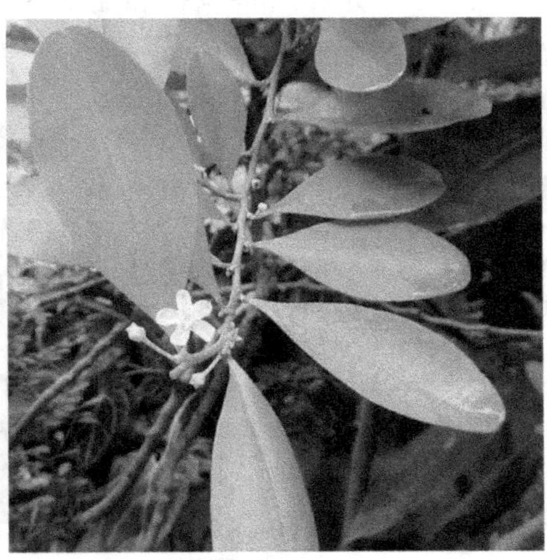

"The chief places for the shipment of Coca are Salaverry - the port of Truxillo in the north, and Mollendo - the terminus of the railroad from the Titicaca region in the south."

"There are two varieties of leaf coming to the North American market: the Huanuco - or large leaf, sometimes referred to as the Bolivian Coca, and the Truxillo - or narrow leaf, known as Peruvian Coca. In selecting a leaf, the several manufacturers with whom I have corresponded have assured me that they base their choice upon the assay and yield of cocaine. For this reason, the Huanuco leaf is the variety commonly found in the market, as it contains a larger amount of cocaine than the Truxillo leaf, which is considered less profitable because of its lower yield of this alkaloid."

## *Truxillo Coca Leaf*

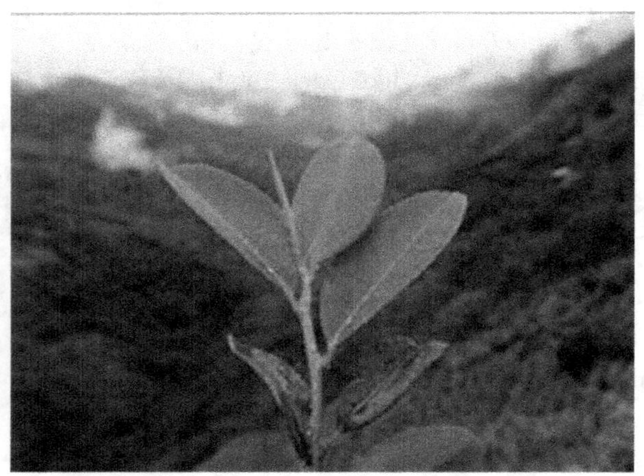

"The native user, however, does not select the hatun-yunca - or large leaf Coca - his choice never being influenced by the amount of cocaine presumably present in the leaf chosen. Locally the distinction is made between hajas dulces - the sweet leaf, and hajas amargas - the bitter leaf, the amount of cocaine present occasioning the bitter quality, while a combination of aromatic principles renders the leaf of more desirable flavor. These principles, though commonly asserted to be exceedingly volatile, are still found in well preserved exported leaves."

"The physiological accounts hitherto published of the action of Coca are often confusional because this distinction in the variety of leaf has not been considered, while many experimenters have contented themselves with enumerating the physiological effects of cocaine rather than that of Coca. In this connection Dr. Kusby says: "In my article I took account of the Bolivian Coca only, which is practically the same as the Peruvian, or Huanuco variety, which is the one used for the manufacture of cocaine. As the leaves are found here in the dried state, their properties are, I believe, almost wholly due to the presence of cocaine, quite different from the properties of the fresh, or very recently dried leaves."

"There is another variety of Coca differing from the Huanuco variety, known as Truxillo leaves, the properties of which as found in this market differ from the Huanuco leaves, while more nearly resembling them in their fresh or recently dried state and as used in the Andes by the natives. You will thus see that all your labors in the direction of physiological research are likely to be fruitless, unless you will be able to ascertain in each case which variety of leaf was used by the one making the report. This I believe to be wholly impossible. Ninety-nine percent of our physicians scarcely know that there are two varieties, or at least that the varieties differ in any way medicinally. The endeavor has been to prevent physicians from learning facts concerning drugs. It is not likely that they can learn from the pharmacist which leaf he used at any particular time, for various reasons."

*Coca Novagranatense*

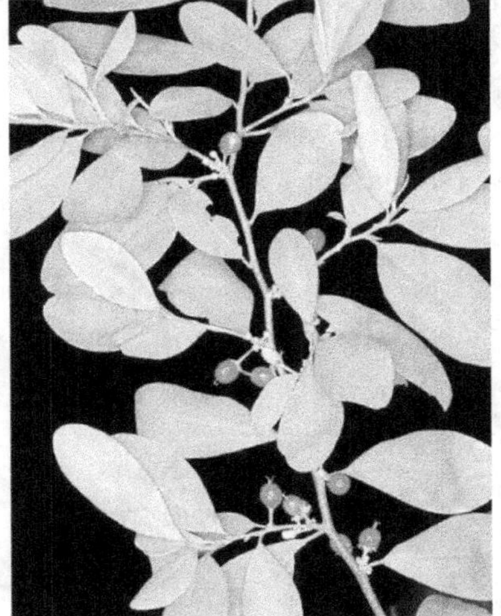

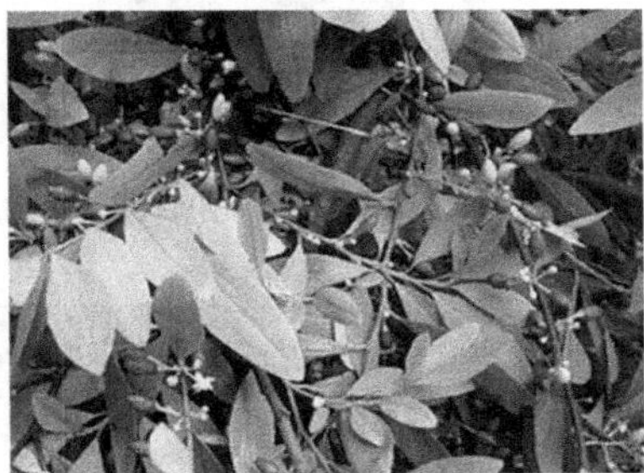

"The biased effort, therefore, to misjudge preparations of Coca because they are not rich in cocaine is but an outgrowth of imperfect knowledge, for the unique quality of the Coca leaf is not solely dependent upon the presence of that alkaloid. It is as Dr. Squibb long since asserted from an intimate study of the qualities of Coca: "But as there is undoubtedly a value to Coca which is not measured by the yield of alkaloid, the proportion of alkaloid does not disprove the alleged inferiority.""

"Thus it will be seen that the Coca leaf as used among the Indians of Peru is one thing, and the variety exported because of its large alkaloidal percentage of cocaine is wholly another matter. This is a distinction which any lover of tobacco will readily appreciate, for surely a fine cigar is never estimated by the amount of nicotine which it contains, nor is the flavor or quality of a delicate tea measured by its percentage of theine."

"We are beginning to learn Coca more intimately and even the more casual observer may soon realize that there is a very wide interim between Coca absolutely inert, as Dowdes well long since would have had us believe: "With less rigor than a whiff of mountain air or a draught of spring water," and the extreme potency which the whole world now recognizes in the alkaloid cocaine."

"The chief interest of Coca to the commercial world has centered upon its possibilities in the production of the one alkaloid, cocaine, instead of a more general economic use of the leaf. Because of this, much confusion of terms has resulted, for chemists have designated the amount of alkaloids obtained from the leaf as cocaine, although they have qualified their statement by saying that a portion of this is un-crystallizable. "

"Numerous experiments have been conducted to determine the relative yield of cocaine from the different varieties of Coca, and when un-crystallizable alkaloids have been found the leaf has been condemned for chemical uses.  It will thus be appreciated how a great amount of error has been generated and continued. The Bolivian or Huanuco variety has been found to yield the largest percentage of crystallizable alkaloid, while the Peruvian or Truxillo variety, though yielding nearly as much total alkaloid, affords a less percentage that is crystallizable, the Bolivian Coca being set apart for the use of the chemists to the exclusion of the Peruvian variety, which is richest in aromatic principles and best suited for medicinal purposes."

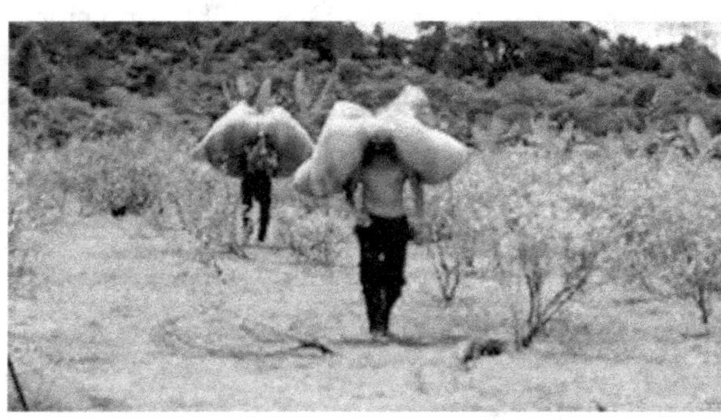

"As a matter of fact, the Peruvian Coca is the plant sought for by the native users. There is not only a difference in the yield of alkaloid from different varieties of Coca, but also a difference in the yield from plants of one variety from the same Cocal, and it would seem possible by selection and propagation of the better plants to obtain a high percentage of alkaloid. At present there is no effort in the native home of Coca toward the production of alkaloid in the leaf through any artificial means."

"Regarding the quality of alkaloid that has been found in the different plants, the Peruvian variety has been found to contain equal proportions of crystallizable and un-crystallizable alkaloid, while the Bolivian variety contains alkaloids the greater amount of which are crystallizable cocaine. Plants which are grown in conservatory, even with the greatest care, yield but a small percentage of alkaloid, of which, however, the un-crystallizable alkaloid seems more constant while the relative amount of cocaine is diminished. In leaves grown at Kew .44 percent, of alkaloid was obtained, of which .1 percent, was crystallizable."

"From experiments of Mr. G. Peppe, of Renchi, Bengal, upon leaves obtained from plants imported from Paris, it was found that leaves dried in the sun yielded .53 per cent, of alkaloid, of which .23 per cent was un-crystallizable. The same leaves dried in the shade on cloth for twenty hours, then rolled by hand, after the manner in which

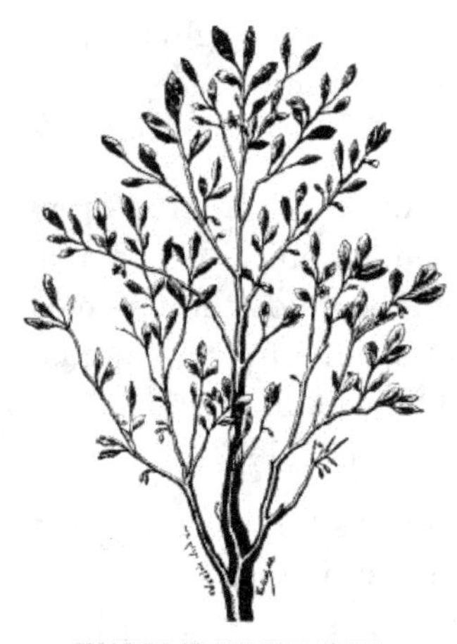

SPECIMEN OF THE COCA SHRUB.

Chinese tea is treated, then cured for two and a half hours and dried over a charcoal fire and packed in close tins, yielded .58 per cent, of alkaloid, of which .17 per cent, was un-crystallizable."

"It is probable that each variety of Coca has a particular range of altitude at which it may be best cultivated. The Bolivian variety is grown at a higher altitude than Peruvian Coca, while the Novo Granatense variety has even been found to thrive at the level of the sea. Among Coca, as among the cinchona certain varieties yield a large proportion of total alkaloids, of which only a small amount is crystallizable."

## Field Descriptions Of Coca

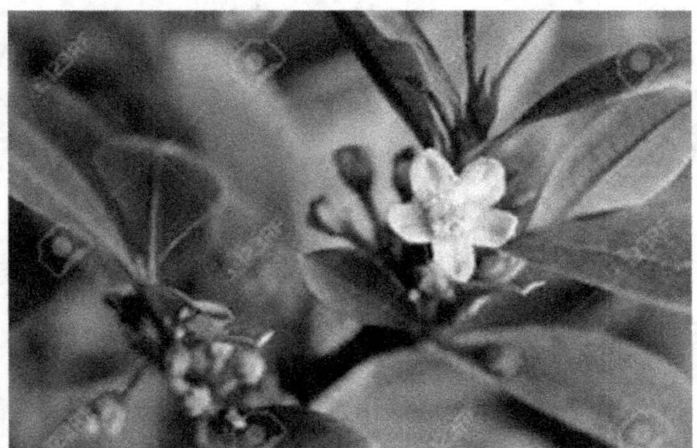

"The Coca tree is easily recognized and, if one finds one's self travelling through the hinterlands of South America or the Far East, or perhaps even Puerto Rico, Algeria or Lebanon, one might do well to keep an eye out for the beauty of Erythroxylon Coca."

"It is a delicate little tree which can upon occasion reach heights of 15-18', but which in fact rarely exceeds 8' in height. Its root system is a large clump of fine rootlets, each terminated by a little tuft of gossamer. The trunk is wrapped in a heavily scored bark, frequently called home by an impressive array of lichen, mushrooms and tiny critters. The lower branches coming off this trunk are few in number; they are alternate on either side, protrude at right angles to the trunk, are occasionally forked and are lightly garnished with leaves."

"The young branches higher on the tree are a pale fern grey. As these branches age they will shift color through a bright green, to a green verging on yellow, and will vary gradually, in the course of ten years or so, then return to the original grey part of the spectrum, finally matching the trunk in color."

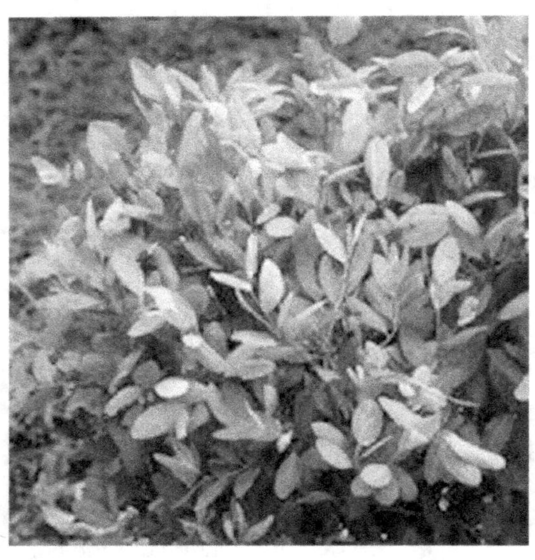

"The leaves are alternate, and are arranged so that their upper faces are always aligned in an orientation with the summit of the tree. The form of the leaves is generally oblong, smooth at the tip and base with a short stem, shaped very much like the leaves of the orange tree. There is a marked darkening aureole effect along the central vein of the leaf. At the base of each leaf one finds a pair of green-brown stipules which are joined together in a roughly triangular shape, and these persist after the leaf has fallen away, leaving a scaly patch for the wound created by the separation."

"The flower buds of Coca nestle against the pitted base of the leaves, and can occur either singly or in groups of as much as ten. The bud is ovoid and with each new push of leaves after a harvest these little clusters - those remaining, that is, on the un-harvested parts of the tree, burst almost immediately into flower. The floral plan is pentametrical, with the petals rising from the base of the bud as a spiral curve with logarythmic proportions."

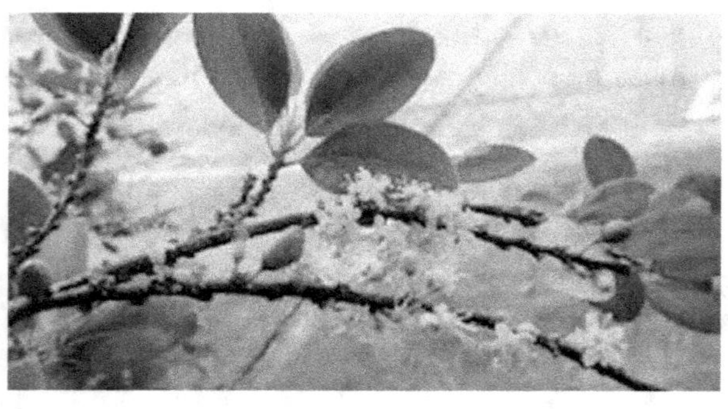

"The flowers are small, delicate and creamy white, and breathe out a faint, sweet aura. The calix is green, and is composed of five sepals, each smooth and pointed, springing from a common base and grandly spread at the summit. The corolla has also five petals, cream-colored, alternate with the sepals, and with the shape of an elongated oval with a faint central nerve showing more on the upper face than on the lower. The corolla falls away immediately after the bloom is full, leaving a naked pistle."

"The stamens number ten, and are pale green filaments of varying length, with the longer ones near the sepals, and the shorter near the flower corolla."

"The stamens rise from the base of the pistle, from inside a small cusp which serves as the nestling place of the ovaries. The ovum are carried within three little wedge-shaped cups within the ovary; after fertilization, all but one of these egg chambers atrophies so that the plant's vital forces can flow undivided into reproduction."

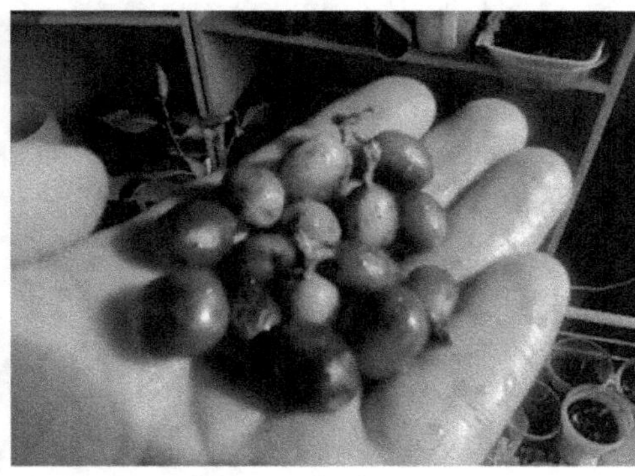

"The new fruit of Coca is pulpy and mucilaginous, a pale green ovoid about a quarter of an inch long, with vestiges of flower adhering to its base. The color of the fruit changes with maturity to a brilliant red, and after fallen and dry it assumes a deep blue-black hue. The seed, only slightly smaller than the dry fruit, is pointed at either end, and is divided longitudinally into six lobes. It is a smooth, pale flesh color. The seed husk is very thin, and the kernel is easily exposed as a hard, white little egg-shaped body."

# Section Three: Traditional Ways Of Growing Coca

## *Ideal Growing Conditions*

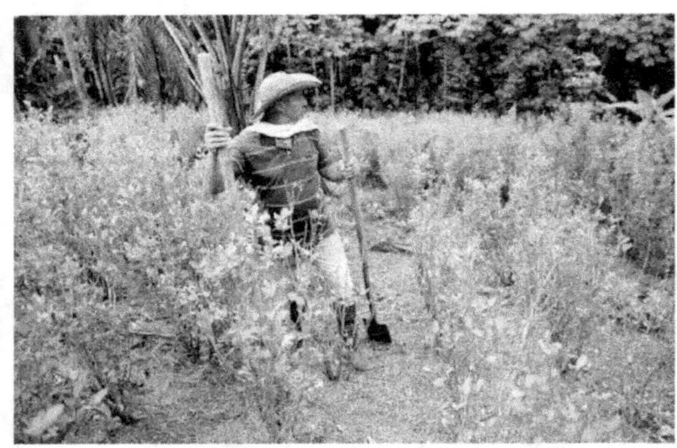

"The temperature in which Coca is grown must be equable, of about 18° C. (61.4° F.). If the mean exceeds 20° C. (68° F.), the plant loses strength and the leaf assumes a dryness which always indicates that it is grown in too warm a situation, and though the leaves may be more prolific, they haven't the delicate aroma of choice Coca."

"It is for the purpose of securing uniform temperature and appropriate drainage that Coca by preference is grown at an altitude above the intense heat of the valleys, and where it is virtually one season throughout the year, the only change being between the hot sun or the profuse rains of the tropical montaña. As the temperature lowers with increase of altitude, when too great a height is reached the shrub is less thrifty and develops a small leaf of little market value, while as only one harvest is possible the expense of cultivation is too great to prove profitable."

"Even close to the equator, in the higher elevations, there is always danger from frost, and for this reason some of the Cocals about Huanuco have at times suffered serious loss. All attempts at Coca cultivation on a profitable scale near to Lima have failed not only because of the absence of rain, but because the season's changing is unsuited."

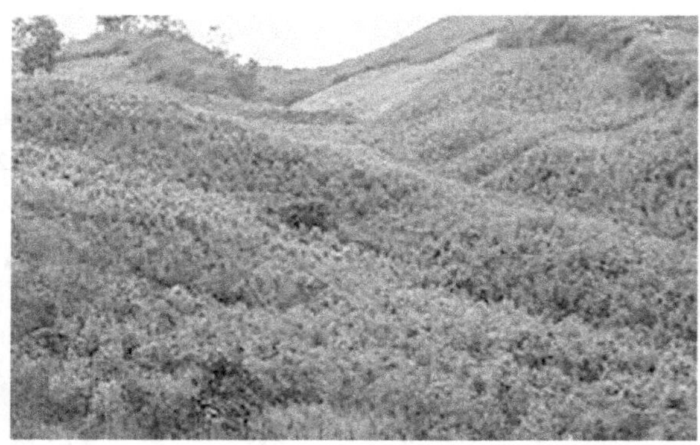

"Coca grows well at altitudes ranging from 1000 to 6000' above sea level. While it grows extremely well at low altitudes, most of the great Coca plantation failures of the 1800s were due to low-altitude planting."

" In Peru Coca grows best and gives the best quality between 700 and 2300 metres; in Sri Lanka successful plantations were 650-800 metres; and in Java from 600-1200 metres. The ideal average temperature for vigorous growth plus leaf quality is 68°F. Coca will not tolerate freezing temperatures in the night or temperatures above 95° for extended periods in the day."

"At the higher part of the temperature range the plant loses much of its vital force, the leaves become dry and the subtle tang of the essential oils is lost. At the lower end of the range the plant becomes dispirited, the leaves remain small, never fully maturing, and the plant cannot be counted on to give more than one lackluster harvest a year."

"While Coca thrives in locations where it receives lots of direct sunlight, it will also do well enough if it must be grown in a relatively shady spot, though it will not show as lush a leaf population at maturity."

"The natural life of the Coca shrub exceeds the average life of man, yet new Cocals are being frequently set out to replace those plants destroyed through accident or carelessness. The young plants are usually started in a nursery, or almaciga, from seeds planted during the rainy season, or these may be propagated from cuttings. In the conservatory slips may be successfully grown if care is taken to retain sufficient moisture about the young plant by covering it with a bell glass."

There seems to be relatively little difference in alkaloid production between shade-grown and sun-grown Coca, though the sparse harvests from the shaded tree do mean significantly less production overall. Coca cannot be effectively cultivated in regions which experience long dry spells, and does best when there is a certain temperate humidity in the air for most or all of the year. It's most important to have a constant, or as nearly constant as possible humidity throughout the year, a situation which bodes well for greenhouse cultivation.

Coca plants don't tolerate overwatering or too much rain – usually not a problem in the high Andes, to say the least. A lot of water makes big, gloriously bushed plants but it literally "waters down" the alkaloid production of the profuse leaves, stranding the grower with a fine harvest of glossy leaves and the prospect of very sore jaw muscles if he is to obtain any of the benefits hoped for in his long efforts. Of course, commercial low-altitude Amazon Coca growers don't care much about leaf quality since they're into extraction not making tea, and security from satellites and airplanes takes precedence over alkaloid quality, and leaf volume more than makes up for hiding under the canopy and tolerating too much rain anyway.

Several ancient writers on the subject of Coca cultivation noted that any area suitable for the growing of Tea or Coffee plants is also eminently suited for Coca cultivation, a fact that might make consultation with your friendly agricultural department a bit less trying if you need assistance in locating a suitable area for any project you might have in mind.

A classic 1983 Harvard Botanical Museum study **https://tinyurl.com/y3sra4ja** says this about Greenhouse Coca:

> *"Light intensity, humidity and moisture availability may influence profoundly the relative leaf size, form, vein thickness and patterns, as well as stomatal and veinlet terminus numbers in all varieties of cultivated coca.*

> *Classical shade-leaf as opposed to sun-leaf structural differences may be found within each variety in relation to microhabitat differences experienced by individual plants and leaves. Humid and shady microhabitat conditions result normally in the development of relatively large, thin leaves with reduced numbers of stomata and veinlet termini per unit area, as well as more slender and less conspicuous veins.*

> *Conversely, sunny and drier habitats induce the formation of small and thicker leaves with comparatively more numerous stomata and veinlet termini, and more prominent, thicker veins. Shade-leaf morphology appears not only in South American coca plants grown under shaded conditions, but also in plants of each variety cultivated under glass at temperate latitudes in North America."*

> *"Aside from an appropriate soil that is well drained, there is another important element to the best growth of Coca, and that is a humid atmosphere. Indeed, in the heart of the Montaña it is either hazy or drizzling during some portion of the day throughout the year, the intense glare of the tropical sun being usually masked by banks of fog, so that it would seem that one living here is dwelling in the clouds. At night the atmosphere is loaded with moisture and the temperature may be a little lower than during the day, though there is usually but a trifling variation day after day."*

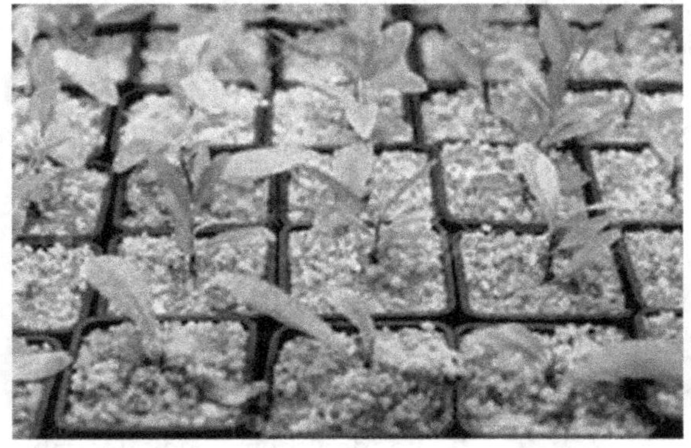

Here's a summary of what many different writers say or hint at regarding the care of Coca seedlings and young plants.

Coca is started like most other plants - by planting the seeds in covered beds which protect the sprouts from the direct sun and from battering rains, not to mention the predations of various creatures. The seeds are traditionally planted one at a time three inches apart. Those selected for planting should be well-ripened, and should be air-dried in a breezy, shaded spot for three days before going into the earth. It is not absolutely necessary to engage in the perhaps perilous business of transplantation; in the higher Andes seeds are generally planted directly into the furrows. In such cases the furrows are covered with a layer of non-acid leaves or with bedding plastic.

Growers say that bedded seeds as well as field-planted seeds should be planted 3/4 inches deep, and should not be watered for several days, and then only sparingly. Culture of Coca requires no special soil other than an adequate supply of humus and sufficient sand/clay to stabilize the soil without loss of permeability.

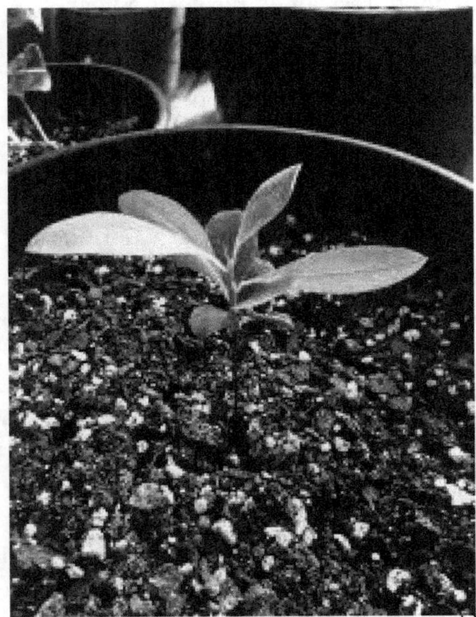

After from two to three weeks the seeds germinate, and one then begins a gradual buildup of exposure of the sprouts to sunlight, at the rate of one hour the first day, two hours the second, and so forth until the sprouts are accustomed to the full daylight cycle in which they will be living. If you don't go through this acclimatization process the little plants will elongate severely and many will topple of their own abnormally stimulated weight, defeated by their Icarus-like reach for the living sun.

During the first six months of their life the little Coca plants are very susceptible to rots and molds, and any infected or infested seedlings should be removed immediately. Also growers check the plants for insect pests regularly during the first six months when they are most vulnerable. After a Coca tree is established it is tough but until then it benefits from regular attention.

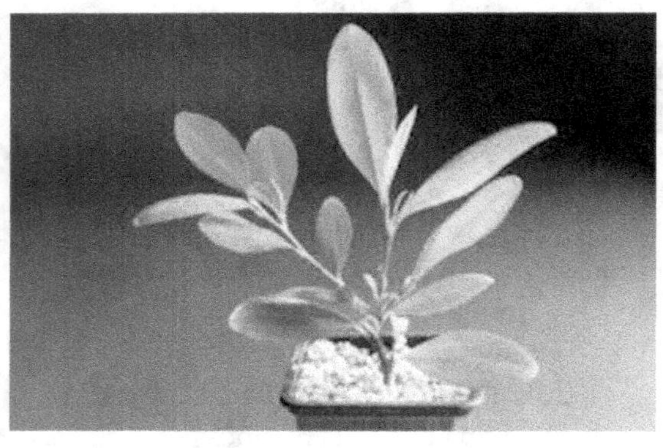

Most writers agree that the seedlings will reach a height of 5" in 8-10 weeks. This is the time to transplant if you have bedded them. They describe taking up a wide, deep ball with each plant and setting them out on rows two feet apart, with the rows themselves spaced at three-foot intervals. Other spacing arrangements mentioned in the literature on Coca planting include plots of 2.5'x 2.5'; 3' x 3'; and in the hill country of the old Java Coca plantations the spacing was 2' x 6'. Java Coca is said to be especially luxuriant in growth and to need lots of space between plants.

After 18 months in the ground it is possible to make the first, most gentle of harvests of young, sweet Coca leaf. The young trees at this point are very tender and can be badly or fatally wounded by a ham-handed harvest. The first harvest is never abundant; however, it marks the beginning of a period when you will be able to obtain several good, restrained harvests a year.

A light harvest stimulates the plant at this and all other points, but with the first effort writers agree that you should take no more than 25% of the leaves, and should leave most of the lower leaves alone. The first harvest must be performed during the dryer part of the year or, in greenhouse cultivation, after a period when the humidity in the air has been gradually drawn down over a period of months.

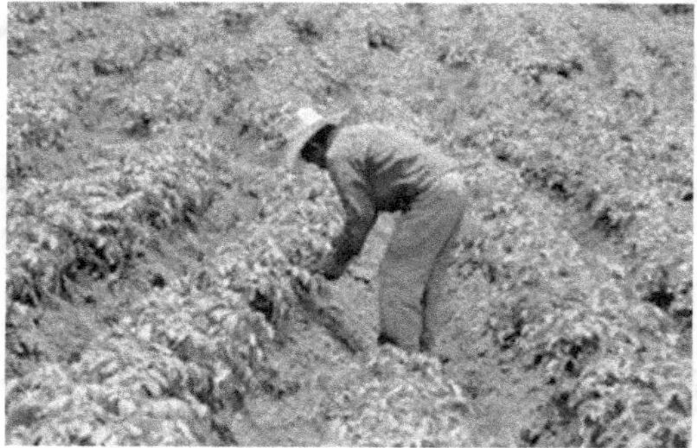

"After this first harvest, the plant is pruned back to a height of one foot above the ground and the lateral branches near the bottom are lightly trimmed back to assist the plant in attaining a solid profile conducive to maximum leaf production later on. The cultivator may expect the equivalent of from four to seven mature leaves from the average plant at first harvest."

"Leaf production and alkaloid strength peak during the 5th-8th years of life, falling off gradually as the plant enters middle age. The Coca of Peru is expected to live for forty years, and this figure seems to hold around the world, though in some places - Java, in particular - the Coca plantations were razed and re-planted every eight years."

"In the fourth or fifth year, when the plants have reached a height of from 3.5 to 4.5 feet, the planters of Peru and Java practiced their first grand harvest, though they harvested carefully and intermittently before that time beginning, as mentioned, at about 11/2 years. Upon occasion one finds planters who make the grand harvest their first, foregoing all previous possible opportunities."

"This seems to be a matter of personal choice and feeling for the state of health of the plant rather than a practice with specific biological basis. In the grand harvest, workers with very sharp, thin-bladed shears pass down the rows of plants cutting each back to a height of 2.5' and trimming back the lower laterals significantly, though not rendering them barren. The yield from such a first harvest on a typical 80 x 80 metre plantation was calculated to be 240 kilos of leaves."

"After the first grand harvest the trees were left to bud and put forth new branches; as soon as these new shoots were well-established, in about six to eight weeks, they were trimmed back once again, before leaf development could begin. With the execution of this second trauma the trees were left alone for six months, and the results were that by the end of their rest period every tree had numerous small, hardy and luxuriant branches, bursting with new leaf."

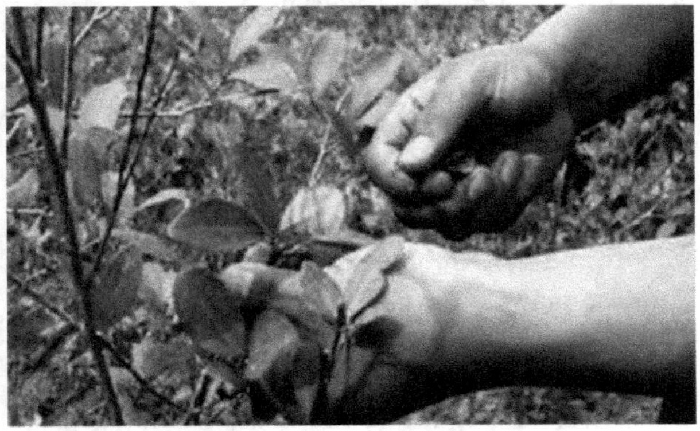

"Beginning, in a sense, with this point in the life of the plant, Coca production can be carried out in earnest. Depending upon the planter harvesting can take place from twice monthly to once every two or three months from this point on. The shorter the period between harvests, however, the more attentive the planter must be to rotating his picking around the needs of his trees - he must pick only a portion of the younger age-groups of leaves. A planter must harvest at least once every three months to prevent his trees from going into seed, thus diverting their vegetative energies from leaf production to seed nurture."

"When an 80 x 80 metre plantation is harvested according to any of the above suggested schedules, the planters expect an annual yield of from 800 to 950 kilos, and the amount doesn't seem to vary much depending on the intervals chosen."

### Early Coca Plant Botany

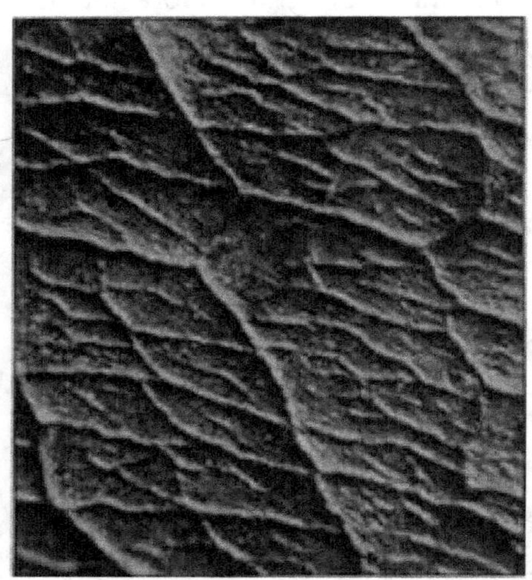

"Some botanists have considered the characteristic lateral lines of the Coca leaf as nerves. Martins was of the opinion these result from pressure of the margin of the leaf as it is rolled toward the midrib while in the bud, the pinching of the tissue causing the substance of the leaf to be raised, resembling a delicate nerve."

"The lines have been designated as "tissue folds" but there is no fold in either the epidermis or substance of the leaf. Histologically the lines are formed by a narrow band of elongated cells, which resemble the collenchyma cells of the neighboring epidermis and serve to stiffen the blade. The lines have no connection with the veins of the leaf and in transmitted light seem like mere ghostly shadows which vanish under closer search."

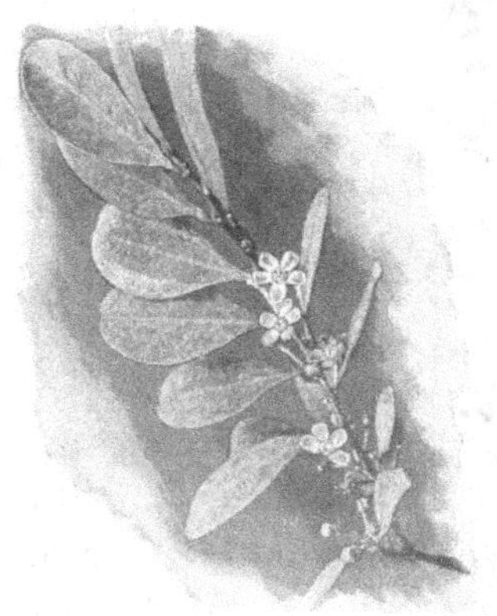

"Many observers have supposed they had found the original locality of wild Coca. Alcide d'Orbigny describes in his travels, having entered a valley covered with what he supposed to be the wild Coca shrub, but thinking he might be mistaken, he showed the plant to his mule driver, who was the proprietor of a Cocal in Yungas, and he pronounced it undoubtedly Coca and gathered a quantity of the leaves. It has been asserted that wild Coca may be found in the province of Cochero, and one of the former governors of Oran, in the province of Salta, on the northern borders of the Argentine Republic, claims to have found wild Coca of excellent quality in the forests of that district."

"Poeppig also described having found wild specimens, known by the natives as Mama Coca, in the Cerro San Cristobal, near the Huallaga, some miles below Huanueo. These examples closely resemble the shrubs of cultivated Coca collected by Martins in the neighborhood of Ega, Brazil, near the borders of the Amazon, and correspond to the wild specimens commonly found throughout Peru."

"In Colombia Humboldt, Bonpland and Kunth described Erythroxylon Hondense as the possible type of the originally cultivated Coca shrub, but there is a difference between the leaves of E. Coca and E. Hondense in the arrangement of their nervures, from which Pyrame de Candolle considers them as entirely distinct species."

"Andre speaks of Coca in the valley of the river Cauca as in abundance in both the wild and half- wild state, but an excellent authority denies that Coca is found wild in Colombia.  The exact locality where Coca is indigenous in a wild state has, however, never been determined. Though there are many Coca plants growing throughout the Montaña outside of cultivation, it is presumed that these are examples where the seeds of the plant have either been unintentionally scattered or else are the remains of some neglected plantation where might have flourished a vigorous Cocal under the Spanish reign. "

"There are evidences of these scattered shrubs throughout the entire region where Coca will grow, but there is no historical data to base a conclusion that these represent wild plants of any distinct original variety, while the weight of testimony indicates that they are examples of the traditional plant which have escaped from cultivation. "

"Coca is indigenous to South America. The different botanists disagree as to which exact family it should be assigned. Linnus, De Candolle, Payer, Raymundi of Lima, Huntk, and others, place it in the family of the Erythroxyleae, of which there exists but one genus, the Erythroxylon, while Jussien adopts another classification and places it in the family of the Malpighiaceae (genus Sethia). Lamarck, on the contrary, believes that this plant should be classed among the family of Nerprem (Rhamnae). In the 21st Century the plant is classified as Erythroxylum coca, but I will refer to it by its historical name throughout this little guide."

"Erythroxylon Coca is a shrub which reaches a height of from six to nine feet and the stem is of about the thickness of a finger. In our climate it cannot thrive except in a hot-house, and there its height does not exceed one metre.

"The root, rather thick, shows multiple and uniform divisions; its trunk is covered with a ridged bark, rugged, nearly always glabrous, and of a whitish color. Its boughs and branches, rather numerous, are alternant, sometimes covered with thorns when the plant is cultivated in a soil which is not well adapted to it."

"The leaves, which fall spontaneously at the end of each season, are alternate, petiolate, with double intra-accillary stipules at the base. In shape they are elliptical-lanceolate, their size varying according to the nature of the plant or of the soil in which it grows."

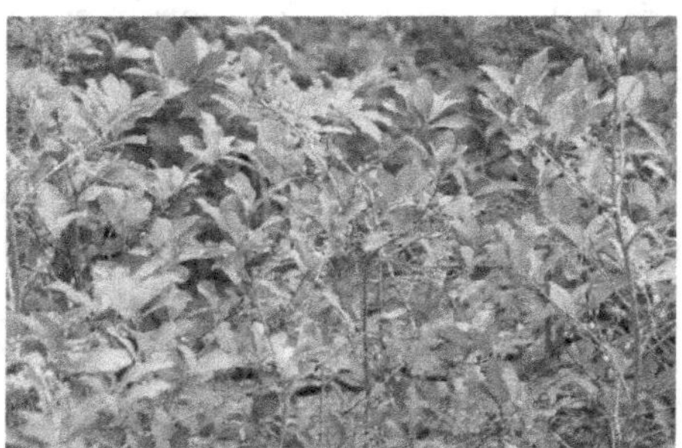

"The leaf of Coca gathered in Peru, of which we give two figures of the natural size, is generally larger and thicker than the leaf of the Bolivian Coca. It is also richer in the alkaloid, consequently much more bitter."

"The Coca leaf from Bolivia, smaller than the Peruvian leaf, is as much esteemed as the latter, although it contains less of the alkaloid. It possesses so exquisite and so soft an aroma, indeed, that the Coqueros seek it in preference to any other."

"The Coca leaves of Brazil and Colombia are much smaller than those of Peru and Bolivia. Their color is much paler. Containing but traces of the alkaloid they are not bitter, and possess a pleasant, but very volatile aroma."

"One of the most important characteristics of the Coca leaf is the disposition of its nervures; parallel with the midrib two longitudinal projections are to be seen, which, starting from the base of the leaf, extend in a gentle curve to its point."

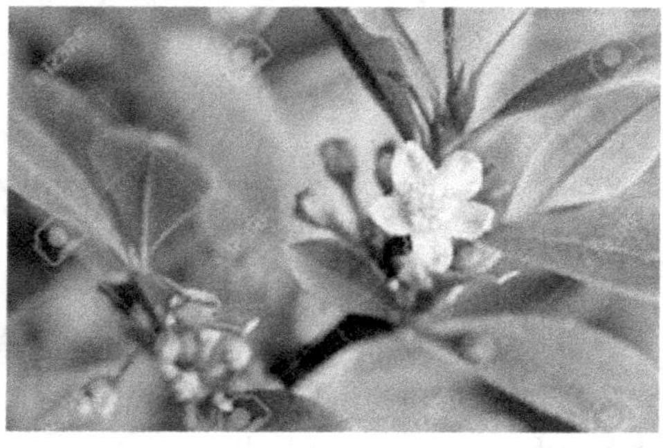

"The exquisite little creamy white flower of Coca is seen in the fields of the Cocals after each harvest, the flowering continuing for about two weeks. The Coca plants which were presented to the New York Botanical Garden have continued to blossom at irregular intervals throughout the year, while M. Mariani told me that the shrubs grown in his conservatories flower in October. The blossoms are very delicate and the petals quickly fall. "

"The upper surface of these leaves is of a beautiful green tint; the lower surface of a paler green, except, however, near the midrib. At this point, there is a strip of green darker than the rest, which becomes brown in the withered leaves."

"The flowers, small, regular and hermaphrodite, white or greenish yellow, are found either alone or in groups in little bunches of cyme at the axil of the leaves or bracts, which take their place on certain branches. The disposition into cymes is that most commonly met with. They are supported by a slender pedicel, somewhat inflated at the top, the length of which does not exceed one centimetre. The sepals, joined at the base and lanceolated, are of a green tint with a whitish top. The petals, half a centimetre in length, pointed, concave inside and yellowish white, exhale a rather pleasant odor."

"They are provided with an exterior appendage, of the same color and of the same consistency, surmounted on each side with an ascending fimbriated leaf, irregularly triangular in shape. The stamens, at first joined in a tube for one-third of their length, afterward separate into white subulated strings, provided with an obtuse ovoid anther which extends a little beyond the petals. The ovary is ovoid in shape and green in color, thickening at the top into a yellowish glandular tissue."

"The style which rises above it separates into three diverging branches, provided with orbicular papilliform bodies at their extremity, obliquely inserted into the slender patina. "

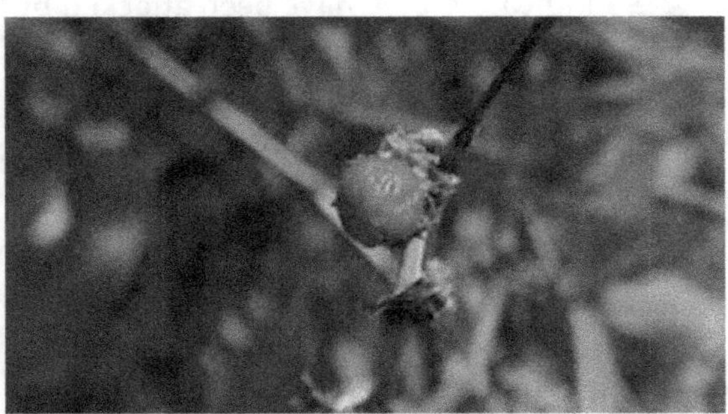

"The fruit is a drupe of an elongated ovoid form, being a little more than a centimetre in length, of a reddish color when fresh, and having a tender, thickish pulp inclosing a seed. This seed shows longitudinal furrows and alternate vertical projections which make its division irregularly hexagonal. When the fruit is dried, the skin assumes a brownish color, shrivels up and molds itself on the protuberances and irregularities of the seed."

"When the fruit has formed it changes color in ripening, through all the hues from a delicate greenish yellow to a deep scarlet vermilion, and upon the same shrub there may be a number of such colorations to be seen at one time.

"Monardes, writing centuries ago, said: "The fruit is in the form of a grape, and as the fruit of the myrtle is reddish when it is ripening, and about of the same dimensions - when attaining its highest maturity becoming darker black."

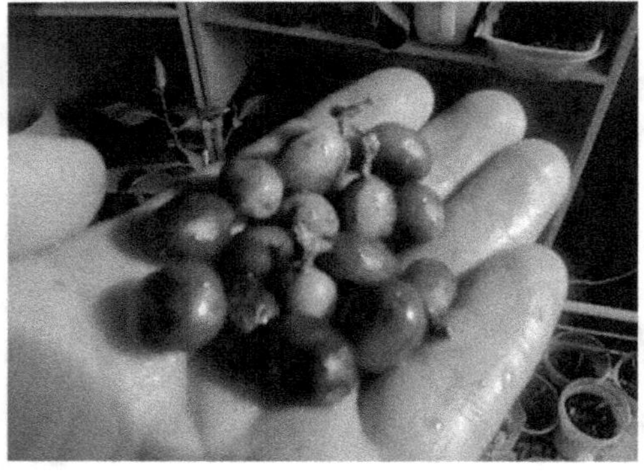

"I was going to say that the fruit resembles the smallest of oval cranberries, both in color and in shape, for I at one time found some little cranberries which appeared so much like the Coca fruit as to seem almost identical; but all cranberries are not alike, and there has already been too much confusion in hasty comparison, so I shall reserve my description for the more technical details. "

"The fruit is gathered while yet scarlet during the March harvest, but if it is permitted to remain on the bush it becomes dark brown or black and shrivels to the irregular lobing of the contained nut."

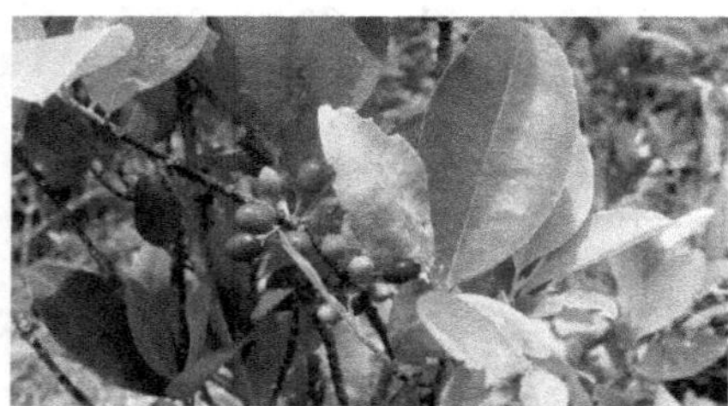

"In selecting the seeds care is taken to cast aside all fruit that is decayed, the balance being thrown into water, and those which are light enough to float are rejected as indicating they have been attacked by insects. The balance is then rotted in a damp, shaded place, to extract the seed, which is washed and sun dried. When it is desired to preserve these any length of time the fruit is exposed to the hot sun, which dries the fleshy portion into a protective coating. But the seeds do not keep well."

"In Peru perhaps they will retain germinating power for about fifteen days, while those from plants grown in the conservatory must be planted fresh, when still red, for if allowed to dry they become useless."

## *Prime Coca Soils Of The Montaña*

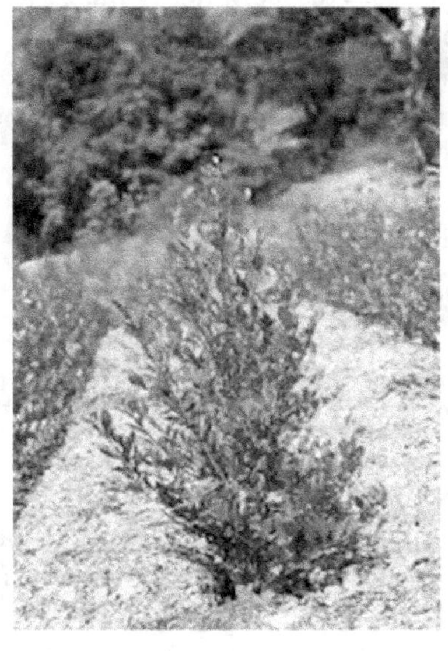

"A peculiar earth is required for the most favorable cultivation of Coca, one rich in mineral matter, yet free from limestone, which is so detrimental that even when it is in the substratum of a vegetable soil the shrub grown over it will be stunted and the foliage scanty. While the young Coca plants may thrive best in a light, porous soil, such as that in the warmer valleys, the full grown shrub yields a better quality of leaf when grown in clay. "

"The clay soil of the montaña affords this property in a high degree, while the hillside cultivation admits of an appropriate drainage the interspaces without which the delicate root would soon be rotted. As the water is absorbed from the soil, a flow by capillarity takes place to that point, and so the Coca root will drain a considerable space."

"The red clay, common in the tropical Andes, is formed by a union of organic acids with the inorganic bases of alkaline earths, and oxides - chiefly of iron which in a soluble form are brought to the surface by capillarity."

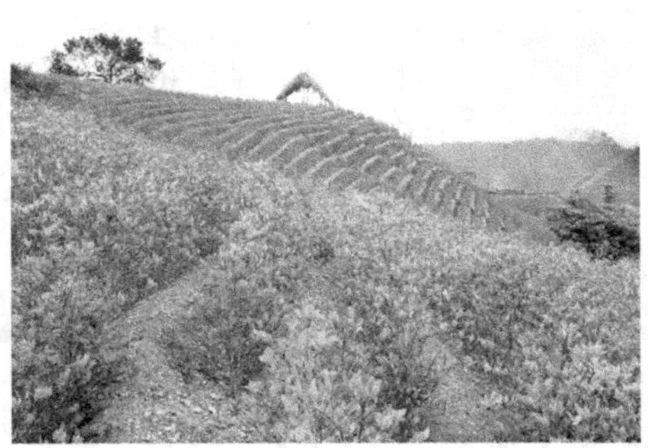

"These elements enter the Coca shrub in solution through its multiple fibrous root, which looks like a veritable wig. The delicate filaments are extended in every direction to drink in moisture, and as these root-hairs enter the interspaces of the soil, the particles of which are covered with a film of water, absorption readily takes place. "

"It is possible a metallic soil may have some marked influence on the yield of alkaloid. At Phara, where the best Coca leaves are grown, the adjacent mountains are formed of at least two per cent, of arsenical pyrites, a fact which is noteworthy because this is the only place in Peru where the soil is of such a nature.

"Most of the soil of the Andean hills where the best Coca is grown, originates in the decay of the pyritiferous schists, which form the chief geological feature of the surrounding mountains. This, commonly mixed with organic matter and salts from the decaying vegetation, or that of the trees burned to make a clearing, affords what might be termed a virgin earth - terre franche ou normale - which requires no addition of manures for invigoration. In the  conservatory it has been found, after careful experimentation, that a mixture of leaf mould and sand - terre de bruyere - forms the best artificial soil for the Coca plant.

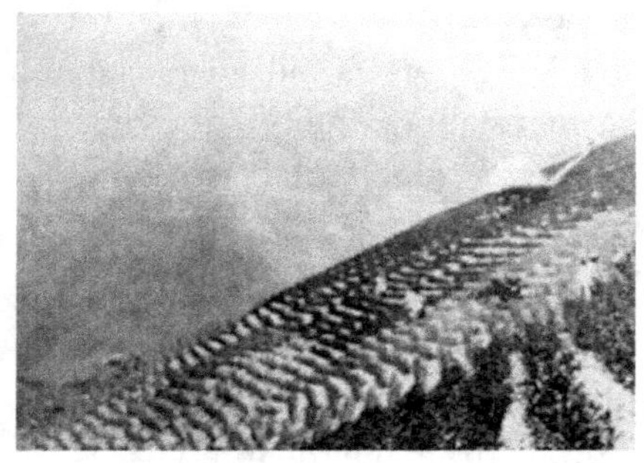

Aside from an appropriate soil that is well drained, there is another important element to the best growth of Coca, and that is a humid atmosphere. Indeed, in the heart of the Montaña it is either hazy or drizzling during some portion of the day throughout the year, the intense glare of the tropical sun being usually masked by banks of fog, so that it would seem that one living here is dwelling in the clouds. At night the atmosphere is loaded with moisture and the temperature may be a little lower than during the day, though there is usually but a trifling variation day after day.

### Coca Seeds & Seedlings Need Protection

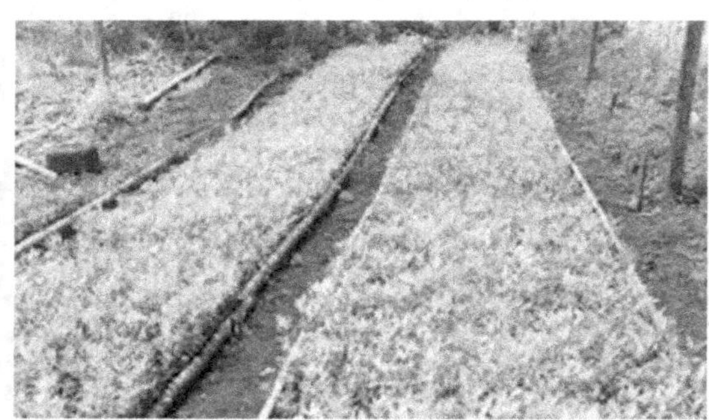

"The birds are great lovers of Coca seeds, and when these are lightly sown on the surface of the nursery it is necessary to cover the beds at night with cloths to guard against "picking and stealing."

"Before sowing the seeds are sometimes germinated by keeping them in a heap three or four inches high and watering them until they sprout. They are then carefully picked apart and planted either in hills or the seeds are simply sown on the surface of the ground, and from that they take them up and set them in other places into earth that is well labored and tilled and made convenient to set them in."

"There is commonly over the beds of the nursery a thatched roof - huasichi - which serves as a protection to the tender growing shoots from the beating rain or melting fierceness of the occasional sun. The first spears are seen in a fortnight, and the plants are carefully nourished during six months, or perhaps even a year until they become strong enough to be transplanted to the field."

## Planting Out Coca Seedlings

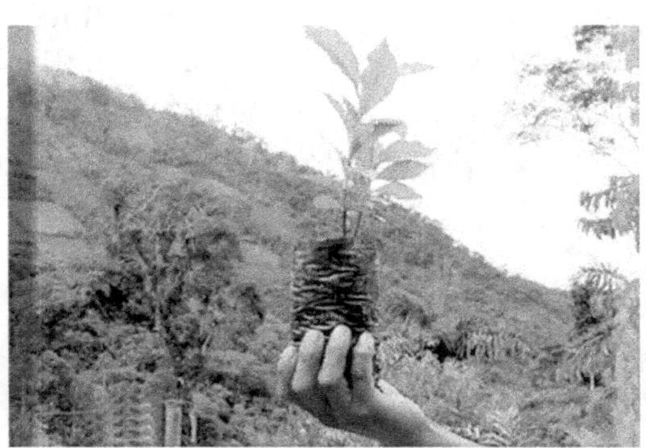

"As a rule, all plants that are forty or fifty centimetres high (16 to 20 inches) may be set out, being placed in rows as we might plant peas or beans. In some cases they are set in little walled beds, termed aspi, a foot square, care being taken that the roots shall penetrate straight into the ground."

"Each of these holes is set about with stones to prevent the surrounding earth from falling, while yet admitting a free access of air about the roots. In such a bed three or four seedlings may be planted to grow up together, a method which is the outgrowth of laziness, as the shrubs will flourish better when set out singly."

"Usually the plants are arranged in rows, termed uachas, which are separated by little walls of earth - umachas - at the base of which the plants are set. In some districts the bottle gourd, maize, or even coffee, is sown between these rows, so as to afford a shield for the delicate shoots against sun or rain."

"At first the young plants are weeded - mazi as it is termed - frequently, and in an appropriate region there is no need for artificial watering: but the Coca plant loves moisture, and forty days under irrigation will cover naked shrubs with new leaves, but the quality is not equal to those grown by natural means."

### The Life Cycle Of A Cocal

"The natural life of the Coca shrub exceeds the average life of man, yet new Cocals are being frequently set out to replace those plants destroyed through accident or carelessness. The young plants are usually started in a nursery, or almaciga, from seeds planted during the rainy season, or these may be propagated from cuttings. In the conservatory slips may be successfully grown if care is taken to retain sufficient moisture about the young plant by covering it with a bell glass."

"As a rule, all plants that are forty or fifty centimetres high (16 to 20 inches) may be set out, being placed in rows as we might plant peas or beans. In some cases, they are set in little walled beds, termed aspi, a foot square, care being taken that the roots shall penetrate straight into the ground. Each of these holes is set about with stones to prevent the surrounding earth from falling, while yet admitting a free access of air about the roots."

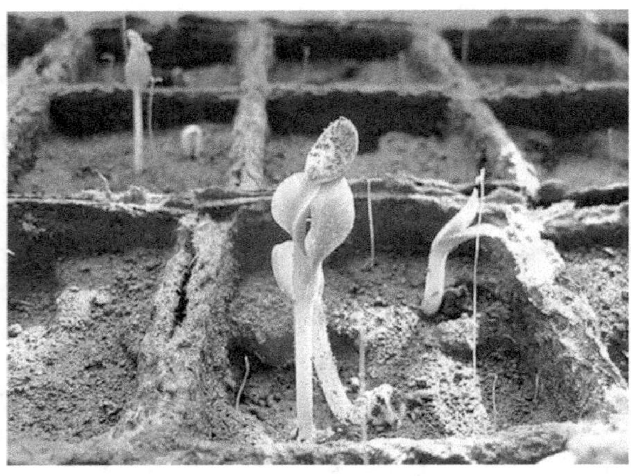

"In such a bed, three or four seedlings may be planted to grow up together, a method which is the outgrowth of laziness, as the shrubs will flourish better when set out singly. Usually the plants are arranged in rows, termed uachas, which are separated by little walls of earth - umachas - at the base of which the plants are set. In some districts the bottle gourd, maize, or even coffee, is sown between these rows, so as to afford a shield for the delicate shoots against sun or rain."

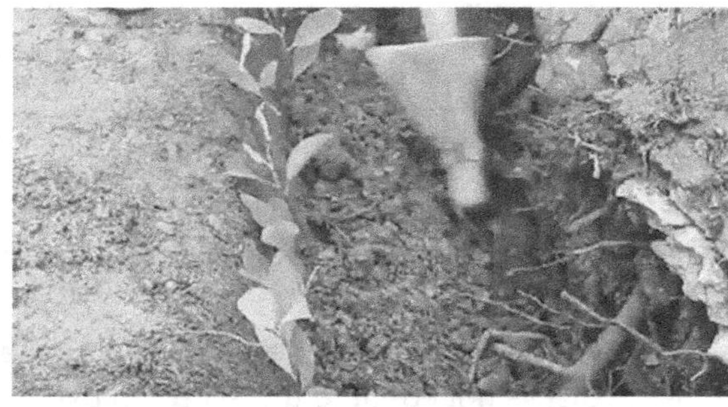

"At first the young plants are weeded - mazi as it is termed - frequently, and in an appropriate region there is no need for artificial watering: but the Coca plant loves moisture, and forty days under irrigation will cover naked shrubs with new leaves, but the quality is not equal to those grown by natural means."

"In from eighteen months to two years the first harvest, or mitta, which literally means time or season—is commenced. The leaves are considered mature when they have begun to assume a faint yellow tint, or better— when their softness is giving place to a tendency to crack or break off when bent, usually about eight days before the leaf would fall naturally. This ripe Coca leaf is termed by the Indians cacha."

"The Coca shrub, growing out of immediate cultivation, will sometimes attain a height of about twelve feet, but for the convenience of picking, cultivated plants are kept down to less than half that height by pruning -

huriar or ecuspar - at the time of harvesting, by picking off the upper twigs,
which increases the lateral spread of the shrub."

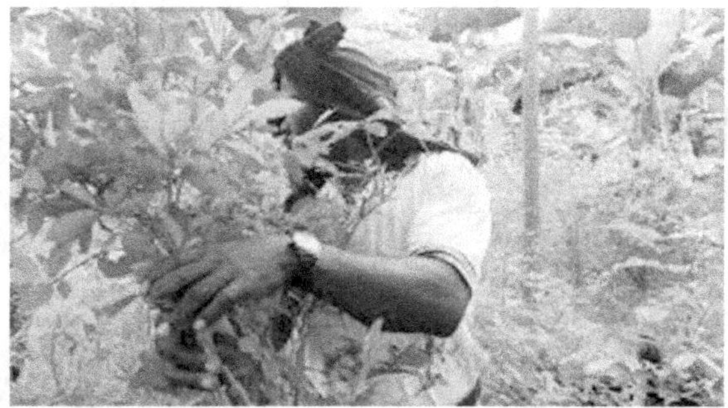

"The first harvest—or rather preliminary picking, is known as quita calzon, from the Spanish quitar—to take away, and calzon—breeches. As the name indicates, it is really more of a trimming than what might be termed a harvest, and the leaves gathered at this time have less flavor than those of the regular mittas. Each of the harvests is designated by name—which may vary according to the district."

"The first regular one in the spring - mitta de marzo - yields the most abundantly. Then, at the end of June, there is commonly a scanty crop known as the mitta de San Juan - the harvest of the festival of St. John – while a third, following in October or November, is the mitta de Todos Santos—the harvest of all saints."

"Usually the shrubs are weeded only after each harvest, and there seems to be a prejudice against doing this at other times, though if the Cocals are kept clear the harvest may be anticipated by more than a fortnight. Garcilasso tells how an avaricious planter, by diligence in cultivating his Coca, got rid of two-thirds of his annual tithes in the first harvest."

# Section Four: All About The Leaf

*Ensuring High Quality Coca Leaves*

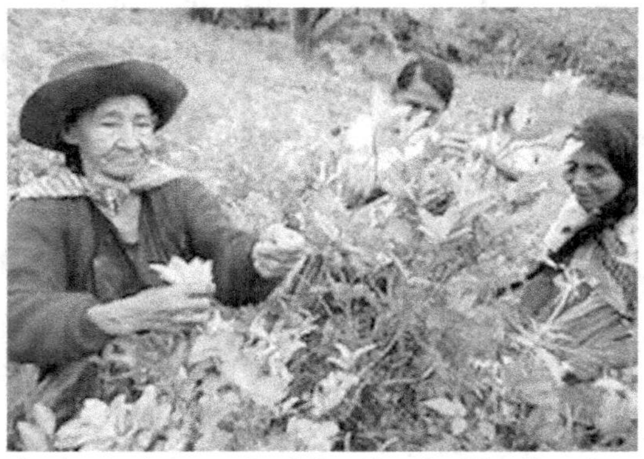

"The Coca shrub, growing out of immediate cultivation, will sometimes attain a height of about twelve feet, but for the convenience of picking, cultivated plants are kept down to less than half that height by pruning - huriar or ccuspar - at the time of harvesting, by picking off the upper twigs, which increases the lateral spread of the shrub. The first harvest - or rather preliminary picking, is known as quita calzon, from the Spanish quitar - to take away - and calzon - breeches."

"As the name indicates, it is really more of a trimming than what might be termed a harvest, and the leaves gathered at this time have less flavor than those of the regular mittas. Each of the harvests is designated by name - which may vary according to the district. The first regular one in the spring - mitta de marzo - yields the most abundantly. Then, at the end of June, there is commonly a scanty crop known as the mitta de San Juan - the harvest of the festival of St. John - while  a third, following in October or November, is the mitta de Todos Santos - the harvest of all saints."

"Usually the shrubs are weeded only after each harvest, and there seems to be a prejudice against doing this at other times, though if the Cocals are kept clear the harvest may be anticipated by more than a fortnight. Garcilasso tells how an avaricious planter, by diligence in cultivating his Coca, got rid of two-thirds of his annual tithes in the first harvest."

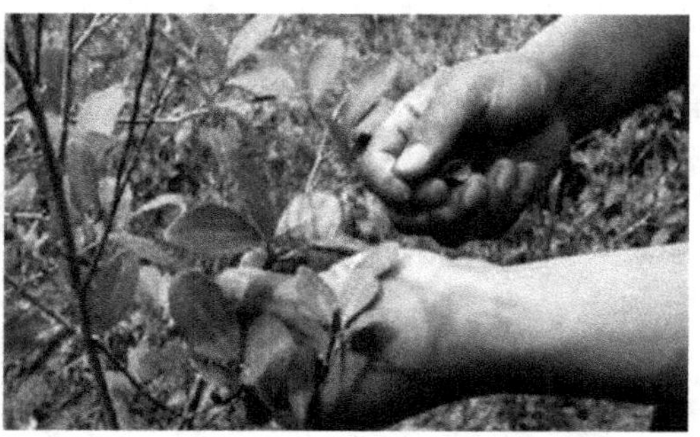

"Picking exerts a beneficial influence on the shrub, which otherwise would not flourish so well. The gathering - palla - is still done by women and children - palladores as they are termed - just as was the custom during the time of the Incas, though the Colombians will not permit women to take part in the Coca cultivation at any time. observer the gathering seems to be done far more carelessly."

"The collector squats down in front of the shrub, and taking a branch strips the leaves off with both hands by a dexterous movement, while avoiding injury to the tender twigs. The pickers must be skilled in their work, for not only a certain knack, but some little force is requisite, as is shown by the wounds occasioned to even the hard skin of the hand of those who are accustomed to the task."

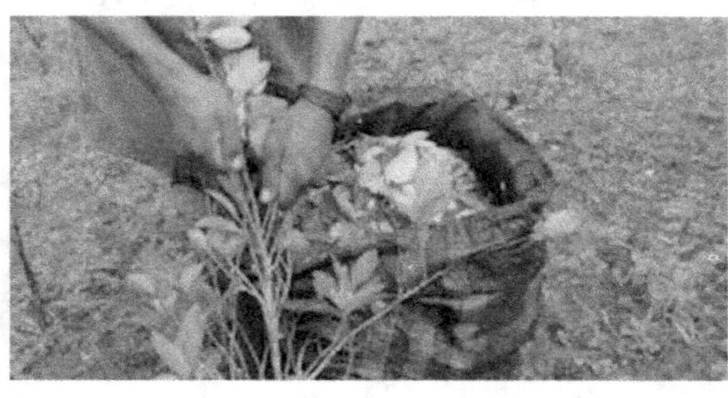

"The leaves are collected in a poncho or in an apron of coarse wool, from which the green leaves - termed matu - are emptied into larger sacks - materos - in which they are conveyed to the drying shed - matucancha. Four or five expert pickers in a good Cocal can gather a cesta- equivalent to a bale of twenty-five pounds, in a day. Harvesting is never commenced except when the weather is dry, for rain would immediately spoil the leaves after they have been picked, rendering them black in color and unsalable, a condition which the Indians term Coca goñupa, or yana Coca."

"Coca when gathered is stored temporarily in sheds - Matuhuarsi - which open into closed courts, the cachi, or matupampa, and the contents of these warehouses indicate the prosperity of the master of the Cocal. In the drying yards of these places the leaves are spread in thin layers two or three inches deep, either upon a slate pavement - pizarra - or simply distributed upon a hard piece of clear ground of the casa de hacienda. The closest guardianship must now be maintained over the leaves during the process of drying, and on the slightest indication of rain they are swept under cover very rapidly."

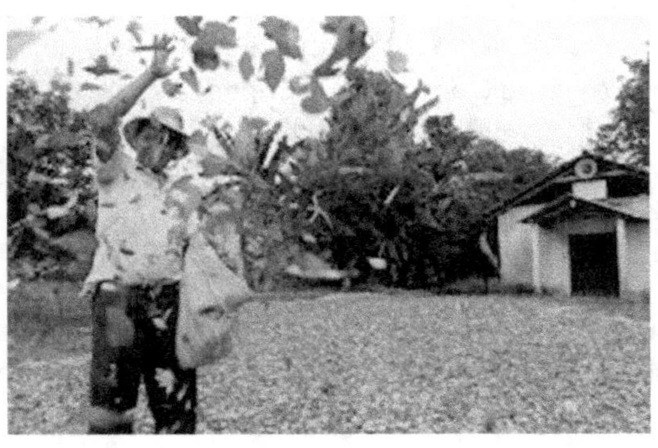

"Drying may be completed within six hours in good weather, and when properly dried under such favorable conditions, the leaf is termed Coca del dia and commands the highest price. A well cured mature Coca leaf is olive green, pliable, clean, smooth and slightly glossy, while those which are old or are dried more slowly assume a brownish green and are less desirable. After drying, the leaves are thrown in a heap, where they remain about three days while undergoing a sort of sweating process. When this commences the leaf is crisp, but sweating renders it soft and pliable. After sweating the leaves are again sun dried for a half hour or so, and are then ready for packing.  If the green leaves cannot be immediately dried, they may be preserved for a few days if care be taken not to keep them in heaps, which would induce a secondary sweating or decomposition and give rise to a musty odor, termed Coca ccaspada which clings even to the preparations made from such leaves."

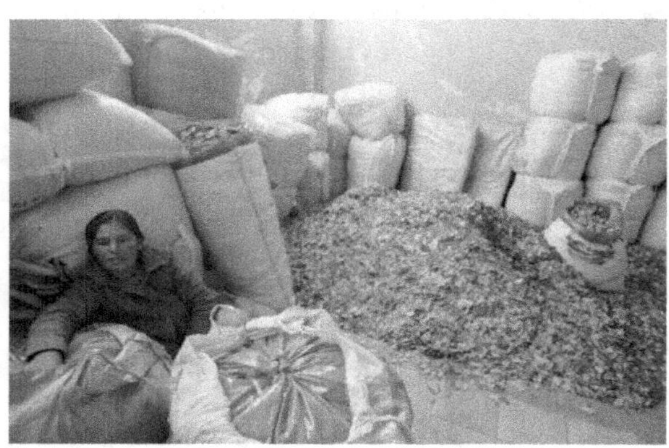

"The refinement of curing maintains a certain amount of moisture in the leaf, together with the peculiar Coca aroma, and it is exact discernment in this process which preserves the delicacy of flavor. When drying has been so prolonged as to render the leaf brittle and without aroma, the quality of Coca is destroyed. It has been suggested that an improvement might be made in drying through the use of sheds, where the leaves could be exposed in layers to an artificial heat, and a current of dry air, after the manner of the secaderos used in Cuba for drying coffee. But whether because of an unwillingness to adopt new methods, or because of some peculiar influence of the atmosphere imparted to the leaf in the native way of drying, all attempts to employ artificial methods have proved unsatisfactory."

## *Distinguishing Quality From Inferior Leaf*

"As in all other details of this research, a variety of expression has been given as to the odor and appearance of the Coca leaf. Doubtless this diversity is due to whether new or old leaves have been examined, or whether the leaves have been suitably dried. Poeppig thought one of the constituents of the  leaves was volatilized by drying, and it is known that the characteristic aroma of the leaf is lost when it is improperly kept."

"The aroma of Coca has been compared to that of about every other thing under the sun, and in one case is actually described as having an odor between hay and chocolate. One can appreciate that it is exceedingly difficult to describe an odor, as the nearest approach to exactitude which may be made is by way of comparison. When it is realized how few people can accurately define the tone from a blending of colors, and when it is considered how much more subtle is the correct perception and interpretation of odors, the difficulty of accurate description may be well understood. "

"Perfumy is an art in which there is a very wide range for expression, which is not only dependent upon the integrity of the observer's sense of perception, but influenced by the temperament of the describer. A freshly opened bale of properly dried and well-preserved Coca has a peculiarly aromatic odor, faintly like vanilla or perhaps suggestive of a finely blended China tea, though more delicate. It has, however, a distinct aroma - the Coca odor sui generis, which once learned can always be readily detected and must afford a means for immediate recognition of true Coca preparations as distinguished from spurious combinations made with cocaine or from poor leaves."

"The Indians select the leaf from its characteristic odor alone, without necessitating even a tasting. This delicacy is only to be preserved by a proper drying and curing, to which end it is considered requisite that the layers of leaves in drying shall be so arranged that the exposure may be uniform to all parts."

"It has been advanced by some writers that the constituents of the Coca leaf are so very volatile that deterioration takes place almost as soon as the leaf has been picked. The Peruvian Indians, however, consider that the leaves may be preserved in their integrity, even in the warm and humid localities where they are gathered, for about a year, and in cooler situations for a much longer time. It has been shown by numerous experimenters that the leaf does not become wholly inert when properly cured and preserved with care, even after several years."

"The leaves examined by Gosse were "the ordinary leaves of commerce, which, though three or four years old, were still greenish and spongy, and possessed characteristic properties."

"Shuttleworth experimented with leaves which had been in his possession for "eight years and yet were still intact."

"Christison used leaves for his physiological experiments which he considered were "at least seven years old," yet because they had been well dried they were still green, flat and unbroken, were bitter to the taste and full of aroma. "

"It may be inferred from these accounts that it is quite possible to preserve Coca leaves in a sound condition for several years if proper precautions have been taken in curing, packing and in their subsequent care."

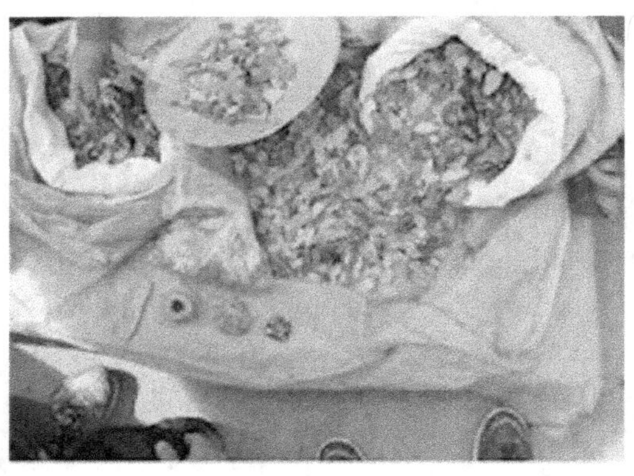

"A conservative estimate as to the yield of Coca throughout South America under an average crop would be from thirty million to forty million pounds per annum, almost this entire quantity being consumed in the countries where it is grown, as a rule, the planters contract with the merchants in town for their whole product, but there is also a retail trade carried on with the country people. Every little Indian village has a fair to its patron saint, and at these there is an interchange of Coca, potatoes, maize and woolen cloths, which may again be sold at a considerable profit. There is possibly left for exportation from one million to one million five hundred thousand pounds of leaves, the value of which varies in accordance with the demand and facilities for transportation. (1885)."

"During the period of 1885-1886, when the newness of cocaine created such an exorbitant price for that alkaloid, Coca was held at thirty-five cents a pound on shipboard at Peruvian ports. Two years ago the leaves were quoted at seven cents a pound at Sandia, while at Asalaya, below Sandia, it was seven pesos and a half, and at Valle Grande, two days further in the Montaña, it was four pesos the cesta - a peso being eighty Peruvian cents, at present equal to about thirty-six cents in United States coin."

"This would make the price of Coca about eleven cents and six cents respectively, varying with the district and subject to fluctuation according to the means of transit. The recent increase of demand for copper has so taxed the means for transportation that the llamas which were ordinarily used for carrying Coca leaves have been pressed into service for carrying copper ore, the result of which has been to advance the price of Coca on the Peruvian coast to twenty cents. Advices from Lima, dated January, 1900, stated that Coca leaves were then held there at twenty-four cents per pound in large lots."

"With the recognition of a volatile principle in the Coca leaf, the proposition was made to solder the packages up in tins like China tea, but this has never been found practicable; in fact, it would be a serious problem to determine the arrangement for carrying such a package, as it should be recalled that the Montaña is hundreds of miles from the coast, to which

Coca can only be conveyed on the backs of mules or llamas in the most primitive way over rugged mountains and through lofty passes, where travel is exceedingly difficult."

### *Traditional Methods Of Picking Coca Leaf*

"The plant begins to yield when it is about a year and a half old. The leaf is the only part of the plant used. It should be gathered in dry weather; this is entrusted generally to women, and simply consists in plucking each leaf with the fingers."

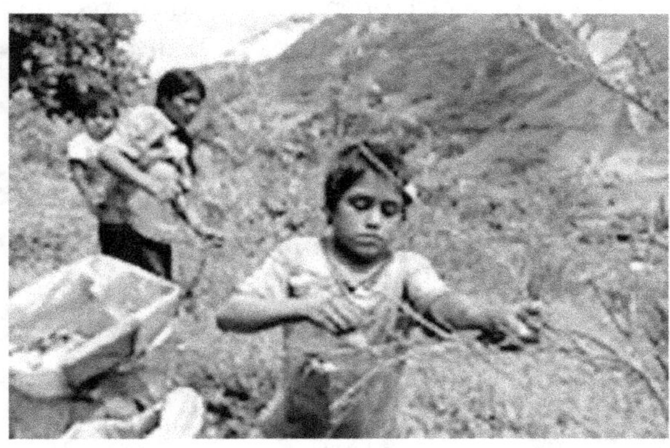

"Picking exerts a beneficial influence on the shrub, which otherwise would not flourish so well. The gathering – palla - is still done by women and children - palladores as they are termed - just as was the custom during the time of the Incas, though the Colombians will not permit women to take part in the Coca cultivation at any time."

"Many writers have spoken of the extreme care with which the leaves are picked or pinched from the shrub, one by one; but to a casual observer the gathering seems to be done far more carelessly. The collector squats down in front of the shrub, and taking a branch strips the leaves off with both hands by a dexterous movement, while avoiding injury to the tender twigs. The pickers must be skilled in their work, for not only a certain knack, but some little force is requisite, as is shown by the wounds occasioned to even the hard skin of the hand of those who are accustomed to the task."

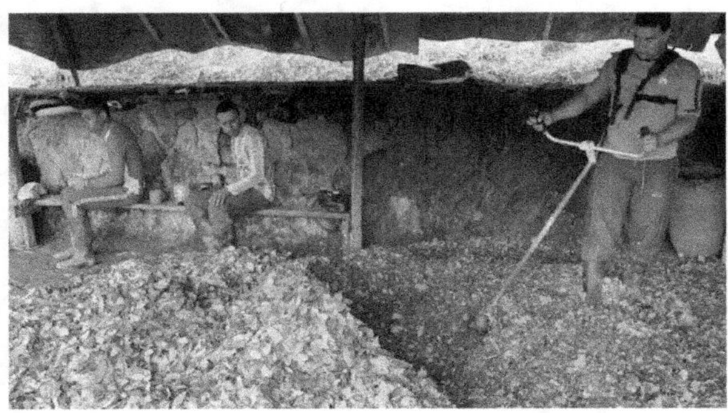

"The leaves are collected in a poncho or in an apron of coarse wool, from which the green leaves - termed matu – are emptied into larger sacks - materos - in which they are conveyed to the drying shed - matucanclia. Four or five expert pickers in a good Cocal can gather a cesta—equivalent to a bale of twenty-five pounds, in a day."

"Harvesting is never commenced except when the weather is dry, for rain would immediately spoil the leaves after they have been picked, rendering them black in color and unsalable, a condition which the Indians term Coca gonupa, or yana Coca."

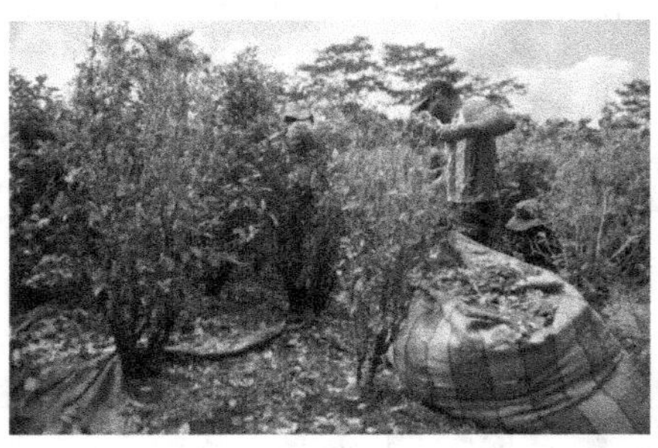

"Coca when gathered is stored temporarily in sheds matuhuarsi, which open into closed courts, the cachi, or matupampa, and the contents of these warehouses indicate the prosperity of the master of the Cocal.  In the drying yards of these places the leaves are spread in thin layers two or three inches deep, either upon a slate pavement – pizarra - or simply distributed upon a hard piece of clear ground of the casa de hacienda."

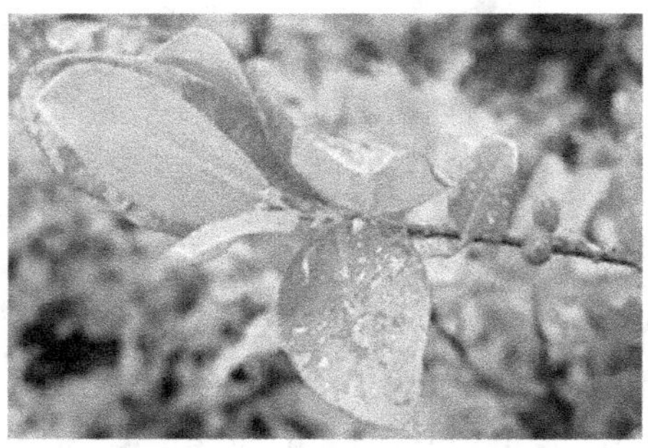

"The closest guardianship must now be maintained over the leaves during the process of drying, and on the slightest indication of rain they are swept under cover by the attendants with the greatest rapidity."

"Drying may be completed within six hours in good weather, and when properly dried under such favorable conditions, the leaf is termed Coca del dia and commands the highest price. A well cured mature Coca leaf is olive green, pliable, clean, smooth and slightly glossy, while those which are old or are dried more slowly assume a brownish green and are less desirable."

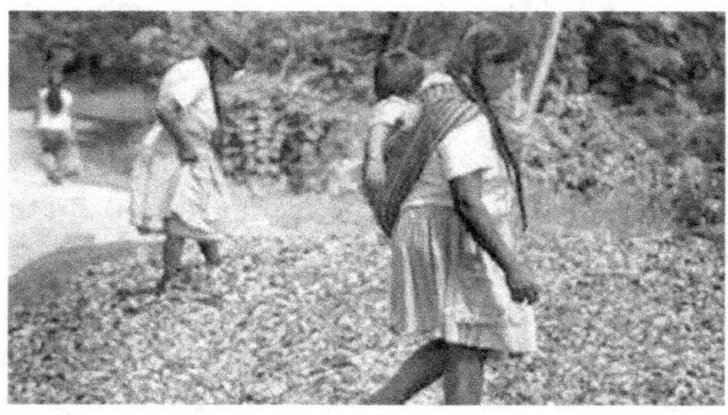

"After drying, the leaves are thrown in a heap, where they remain about three days while undergoing a sort of sweating process. When this commences the leaf is crisp, but sweating renders it soft and pliable. After sweating the leaves are again sun dried for a half hour or so, and are then ready for packing."

"If the green leaves cannot be immediately dried, they may be preserved for a few days if care be taken not to keep them in heaps, which would induce a secondary sweating or decomposition and give rise to a musty odor, termed Coca cespada, which clings even to the preparations made from such leaves.

"The refinement of curing maintains a certain amount of moisture in the leaf, together with the peculiar Coca aroma, and it is exact discernment in this process which preserves the delicacy of flavor. When drying has been so prolonged as to render the leaf brittle and without aroma, the quality of Coca is destroyed."

"It has been suggested that an improvement might be made in drying through the use of sheds, where the leaves could be exposed in layers to an artificial heat, and a current of dry air, after the manner of the secaderos used in Cuba for drying coffee. But whether because of an unwillingness to adopt new methods, or because of some peculiar influence of the atmosphere imparted to the leaf in the native way of drying, all attempts to employ artificial methods have proved unsatisfactory."

"We quote from the Voyage dans la region du Titicaca, by Paul Marcoy, the following passage (" Tour of the World," May, 1877): "Of all the valleys of the Carabaya group, Ituata is the one where Coca is cultivated on the largest scale. They were then at the height of the work, peons and peonnes were following each other through the plantations of the shrub, so dear to the natives that a decree of 1825 placed it in the crown of the arms of Peru, alongside of the vicunia and cornucopia, or horn-of-plenty. Men and women carried a cloth slung across the shoulders in which were placed the leaves, as they gathered them one by one. These leaves, spread out on large awnings, were exposed to the sun for two or three days, then packed up in bags of about one metre in size and sent off to all parts of the territory."

"This gathering of the Coca is just such an occasion for rejoicing for the natives of the valleys, as reaping-time and harvests are for our peasants. On the day when the gathering of the leaves is finished both sexes that have taken part in the work assemble and celebrate, in dances and libations, the pleasure they experience in having finished their labors."

## *Harvesting For Maximum Purity & Potency*

"The plant commences to give its first crop at the end of about one year and a half. The gathering must be done in dry weather; it is generally confined to women, and consists simply in detaching each leaf with the fingers. The leaves are collected in aprons, stored with care under awnings or in bags, sheltered from rain and dampness, dried, and then packed."

"We quote from "Voyage in the Region of the Titicaca," published in "Around the World," May, 1877: Of all the valleys of the group of Carabaya, Ituata is the one where the Coca is cultivated on the largest scale. Were then in full harvest; peons and peonnes followed each other through the plantations of that shrub, so dear to the natives that a decree of 1825 had it placed in the coat of arms of Peru, together with the vicuna, and the cornucopia or horn of plenty. Men and women carried, slung over their shoulders, cloths in which were placed the leaves they had gathered one by one."

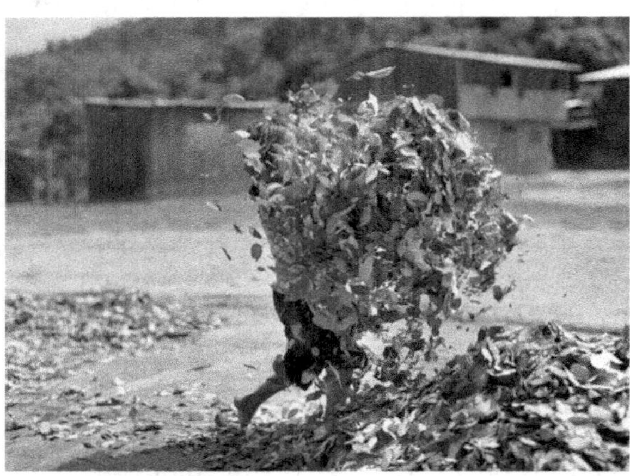

"These leaves, spread out on large mattings, were exposed to the sun's rays for two or three days, and then packed up in bags of about one metre in size, and sent over the entire territory. This harvesting of Coca is for the natives of the valleys an occasion of great rejoicing, as is for our farmers their harvest and vintage time. Oh the day when all the crop is gathered in, both sexes meet, and celebrate it by dancing, drinking, and various sports."

"If the cultivator has only a few trees for personal use, chances are that he will not be engaged in production of any finished product but, rather, will simply follow the time-honored consumption ritual of the coquero, who, whenever the spirit moves him, plucks a fresh leaf or two and chews. On the Coca plantations, however, the Coca is intended for further processing and is treated in the following manner."

"The fresh leaves are spread evenly and thinly on flat metal trays. Clumps of leaves are broken up, and care is taken to assure that each leaf has maximum exposure to the air. With this precaution, fermentation and mould-formation can be avoided. Either of these problems causes great trouble as odor, color and strength will be adversely affected. The leaves are laid out on their drying pans in warm, windy shade on a hot, dry day. "

"They are never exposed to the direct sun in drying. If they are being dried artificially the heat must be blown across them at a point no greater than 120°F., with plenty of fresh-air ventilation. There are a number of studies showing a drop in effective alkaloid content of from .34% by weight in the fresh state to .14% by weight after exposure to the direct sun for only three hours."

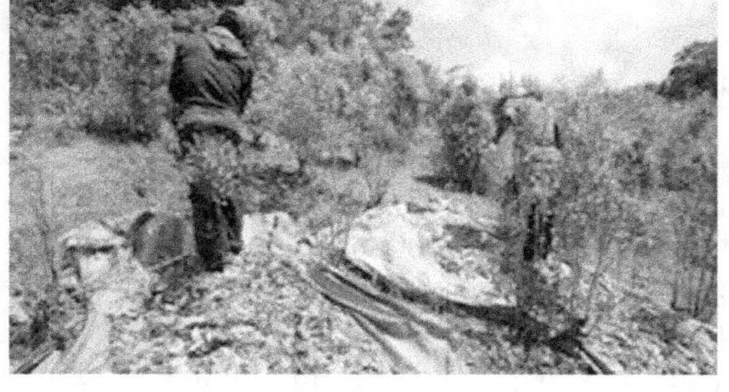

"Whatever the process used, the leaf is considered dry when it can be broken cleanly by bending slightly, and the average time for drying in a hot, dry environment is from 36 to 40 hours. Needless to say, the leaves must be protected from nighttime moisture."

"The dried leaves are taken and pulverized - the devices used vary from area to area. The powder obtained should be uniform, and should be immediately placed in airtight containers. This powder then forms the basis for further processing into refined Cocaine. "

## Section Five: Mama Coca & The Invaders

The discovery that Coca leaves could be refined into yielding their Cocaine really was the beginning of the end, at least of Coca Leaf as a natural medicine. As soon as people experienced straight Cocaine they no longer had any use for Coca leaf – they went directly for the hard stuff, as people will always do. Look at what has just (2019) happened to Cannabis flowers in the few years since broad legalization. A global Cocaine epidemic followed for the next hundred years or so, then paused for a couple of decades, then came back full force with Crack Cocaine in the 1980's. Coca Leaf tea has been rather overlooked in all the commotion.

The same is happening with Cannabis. Before legalization people treasured whole Cannabis flower buds. In most places they were rare and expensive, and people appreciated them and lingered over them like a bottle of very nice wine or a great meal with a loving companion.

Then came 'legalization' and almost overnight people were extracting THC and dressing it up in all kinds of appealing forms and marketing it as a quick and easy high, no mess involved, and so cool all your friends are into it. People just walked away from the Cannabis flower and toward the bright lights as if entranced – behavior so predictable that it's money in the bank. It has worked every time in history a new pleasure has been discovered or invented, and it worked with Coca Leaf and Cocaine just like it's working today with Cannabis Flowers vs. THC extracts, and Tobacco vs. Nicotine vapor.

But things coming full circle also happens so I fully expect that individual Coca growing will begin happen in many places in the world (no doubt already is), and that Coca Leaf will become known again as a powerful natural medicine. Certainly not the only one, or somehow the 'best' one, but certainly a gift from the Great Spirit or, as she is known, Mama Coca.

Since the purpose of this book is to gather together and share as much interesting and relevant Coca knowledge as possible, I'm hoping that the tidbits I've gathered together in this second section will also interest you. Whenever possible I've printed the hyperlink to the original source so that you can follow it if you wish.

## *Return Mama Coca To Her People*

People of conscience rightfully condemn the Nazi looting of art and cultural artifacts from Jewish victims of the Holocaust, and from homes and museums around Europe. People also rightfully condemn the berserk destruction of cultural and historical treasures in Iraq and Afghanistan by ISIS and the Taliban. Many people also have living memories of colonial genocide and cultural looting of the European empires.

There is a growing body of international law that condemns and demands reparations on the part of former colonial powers like Britain, France, Belgium and The Netherlands whose military and "explorers" looted cultural and historical treasures of Greece, Egypt, Iraq, India, Indonesia, Africa and elsewhere in their Empires. The Spanish are certainly near the top of any list of looters of cultural and historical artifacts with their centuries-long conquest and domination of the Indian civilizations of Latin America.

And of course it can hardly be disputed that the Americans top the list of looters with their genocide against Native Americans and blatant theft of their ancient homelands, along with widespread looting of their cultural and historical artifacts, desecration of their graves, and theft of their cultural heritage. When this history is combined with the destruction and enslavement of entire African civilizations, and the forced obliteration of not only whole families and tribes but whole histories, Americans are definitely at the top of any list of historical and cultural criminals.

All of the victims of these various exercises of colonial avarice, hatred and slaughter are at some stage in seeking reparations. The Greeks want their temples back from the British. The Egyptians want the bones and treasures of their ancient Kings returned. Native Americans are demanding the return of their sacred objects and the bones of their ancestors from the Smithsonian. The Iraqis who have seen their Mesopotamian heritage scattered to the winds for centuries are currently being victimized by a blow-dried reincarnation of Jim & Tammy Faye in the person of the "Christian" owners of the tacky little "Hobby Lobby" chain in the US that is charged with large-scale looting on ancient artifacts in the Middle East. These elaborately coiffed smiley-face Oklahoma faux-Jesus worshipers of course deny everything, pleading that they had no idea that these little ole' tiles were invaluable cultural artifacts.

Cultures worldwide are demanding the same of museums in France, Belgium and The Netherlands. The Chinese are demanding the return of cultural and historical treasures looted by the American-backed Chiang Kai Shek. American Black people are demanding reparations for the theft and brutalization of their families, cultures and history. Latin American cultures are demanding that Spain , Portugal and the Catholic Church return the wealth in gold, silver, culture and history stolen from them over the centuries of Colonial domination.

However, in the midst of all this worldwide outcry against theft of cultural and historical heritage by force and stealth, at least one enormous crime against Native People has been completely overlooked, and I am proposing that the people of Bolivia and Peru, who are the victims of this particular crime, organize and pursue legal remedy under the same body of international law that has begun to recognize the rights of other Native People worldwide.

The crime I am referring to is the theft of the Coca Plant by the European pharmaceutical industry that, since the 1840's, has made hundreds of billions of dollars from the theft of this Sacred Plant of the Incas and has not paid one penny in reparation or shared any of the huge profits that this industry has enjoyed for over 150 years. Specifically, I am suggesting that Bolivia and Peru jointly sue the German Pharmaceutical company Merck, which was responsible for first looting Coca Plants from Bolivia and Peru and then extracting the alkaloid Cocaine from those plants, and then making Cocaine the core of the company's fortunes as it grew into the globally dominant pharmaceutical giant of today.

The Coca Plant is indigenous to only one place in the world – the southern Andes – so Merck cannot claim that they took a plant that was readily available worldwide and simply exercised their scientific genius in producing Cocaine. The plants that Merck used to create mountains of gold from a few green leaves came from only one place, and were the cultural and historical heritage of only one People – the Native peoples who today live in poverty in Andes, remote from even a handful of the wealth so jealously guarded by the German pharmaceutical industry and others worldwide who profit from the cultural heritage of the Incas – companies like Coca Cola, who should also be named in any lawsuit for reparations brought by representatives of the Native People of Bolivia and Peru.

The art looted by the Nazis is being returned to the rightful owners under the law, and the families and descendants of those owners are rightfully being compensated. The stolen art, artifacts and bones of ancient civilizations in Greece, Egypt and elsewhere are gradually being pried loose from the talons of the museums erected by Colonial powers to display their loot. Even the American Smithsonian is finally, reluctantly recognizing that it has no right to make the corpses of Native Americans part of their "display", and are, while doing a lot of foot-dragging, gradually returning the bones and cultural and historical loot stolen from the Native American people. And although there is enormous opposition among the elite and their toadies toward paying reparations to American Black people, at least there is some movement among American Black people themselves to reclaim parts of their stolen cultural and historical heritage.

So why shouldn't Merck, Coca Cola and others that have profited from the theft of the heritage of the Incas be taken before the bar of international justice and stripped of at least a major portion of the profits that they have made from the theft of the cultural/historical heritage of the descendants of the Incas? The court of jurisdiction would also be responsible for assuring that the money recovered in the name of the descendants of the Incas was not re-looted by politicians in those countries, and instead went into a closely supervised non-profit international organization that was capped in the top salaries it could pay and the administrative overhead it could charge.

I think that this is the right thing to do, and I think it should be done beginning now. The indigenous People of the Andes have an historic opportunity to force the greedy capitalists of Merck, Coca Cola and other evil corporations to crawl on their knees dragging wagonloads of stolen wealth back to the people who are its rightful owners.

### *Coca Here, Coca There … Coca Alkaloids Everywhere*
Nature, in this spiritual incarnation Mama Coca, never makes something only once. Replication is the name of her game. Make enough copies in enough places and some will survive and of those some will thrive. Everything will try to reproduce, and even some low forms may accidentally make a high form, so that's all good, but high forms that manage to reproduce tend to create more high forms, which suits Mama Coca just fine. Mama likes diversity.

Cocaine and other beneficial alkaloids have been found in varying concentrations in dozens of species of genus Erythrolylum, not just in e. Coca, the great Coca plant of the Andes most closely associated with Cocaine production. These other wild species, some of which are alkaloid-rich. are broadly distributed in South America and may well be more widespread. They could be in your neighborhood plant nursery for all we know. What we do know is that Harvard scientists found Cocaine in 51 species of plants, all from old and probably dusty museum collections. Most of them only had small concentrations of Cocaine, and had varying concentrations of other important alkaloids, but several were more than just mildly Cocaine-rich.

But the real "Wow!" factor to me in all this Harvard research is that there are wild species of the genus Erythroxylum scattered around the world with many of the alkaloids and other good stuff that provide the well-documented health benefits of the Erythroxylum Coca of the Andes. While the authors of this study found that almost all of the wild species that contained Cocaine had very small amounts, you have to wonder what a little tender loving cultivation would do to the alkaloid content of at least some of these wild species? I hope that some folks are already familiar with this study and are already growing Erythroxylum species in greenhouses and working on whatever needs to be done.

This very interesting paper sheds light on the diversity of:

***"Cocaine Distribution In Wild Erythroxylum Species"***

*https://tinyurl.com/y3z92vt9*

"Cocaine distribution was studied in leaves of wild Erythroxylum species originating from Bolivia, Brazil, Ecuador, Paraguay, Peru, Mexico, USA, Venezuela and Mauritius. Among 51 species, 28 had never been phytochemically investigated before. Cocaine was efficiently and rapidly extracted with methanol, using focused microwaves at atmospheric pressure, and analysed without any further purification by capillary gas chromatography coupled to mass spectrometry. Cocaine was reported for the first time in 14 species. Erythroxylum laetevirens was the wild species with the highest cocaine content. Its qualitative chromatographic profile also revealed other characteristic tropane alkaloids. Finally, its cocaine content was compared to those of two cultivated coca plants as well as with a coca tea bag sample."

In 1983 two other American investigators "detected trace amounts of cocaine in 13 neotropical wild Erythroxylum species representing five sections of the genus, and they found that two species from Venezuela, namely Erythroxylum recurrens and Erythroxylum steyermarkii, contained cocaine amounts "comparable to those found in cultivated species." Erythroxylum laetevirens looks more like a vine than like a Coca bush but it apparently produces the Cocaine alkaloid like a champ.

*You can find the E. laetevirens report mentioned above at:*
*https://tinyurl.com/yytbvozj*

It appears to grow wild all over Central and Western Brazil. I'm told that it is a well-known herb and must be gathered carefully.

Harvard scientists only tested decades-old leaves of wild species, but another group tested contemporary Coca Leaf Tea products from Bolivia and Peru. Their findings should encourage anyone who is interested in using these readily available (in Bolivia and Peru) commercial products for dealing with health issues because the researchers conclude that some of the products sold in Bolivia and Peru are "pure Coca leaf" and others, even the "de-cocainized" products that are sold in the US (check Amazon), not only are not completely "de-cocainized" but they appear to still have a leaf chemistry profile that indicates the good quality teas might be somewhat effective as medicinal beverages.

***Here's that interesting study of the alkaloid content of current Peruvian and Bolivian Coca Leaf teas.***

*https://tinyurl.com/yyky8oey*

Coca Teas available in the US are definitely not pure, natural whole Coca Leaf thanks to the War on Drugs, but maybe they are not altogether useless either. It appears that some of the commercial Coca Leaf teas produced in Bolivia and Peru are pure, natural Coca Leaf – the way the great spirit of Mama Coca made them.

***Check out some very interesting research on Cocaine in Coca Teas at:***

*https://tinyurl.com/y3hk7886*

Finally here's an analysis done by the US DEA in 2004 on a selection of Coca Leaf medicines, nutritional supplements and other Coca products from the open market in Bolivia and Peru.

| Product | Treatment | Matrix | µg/mg Cocaine |
|---|---|---|---|
| Ron Fernando Ron De Coca | liquor | Alcohol | 0.22 |
| Ajayu de Coca Pachamama | liquor | Alcohol | Not detected |
| Adelgazante | Diet | Aqueous | 0.39 |
| Anti Diabetico | Diabetes | Aqueous | 0.15 |
| Tos Asma | Asthma | Aqueous | 0.29 |
| Prostata | Prostate Problems | Aqueous | 0.38 |
| Parasitos | Parasites | Aqueous | 0.33 |
| Ulceras | Ulcers | Aqueous | 0.01 |
| Tonico | Tonic | Aqueous | 0.26 |
| Pomada Natural de Coca Contra Dolores: Reumaticos, Musculares, Varices Y Huesos | rheumatic, muscular, veins, and bones | Wax | 0.07 |
| Pomada Natural de Coca Para: Artritis Y Gota | Cream for arthritis and foot pain | Wax | 0.10 |
| Pomada Natural de Coca Para: Hemorroides | Cream for hemorrhoids | Wax | 0.04 |
| Pomada de Molle | Cream for moles | Wax | 0.01 |
| Chicle Cocaplus | Chewing gum | Candy | 0.01 |
| Caramelos Y ElixirEnergizante de Altura | Caramel candy for energy booster | Candy | 0.003 |
| Mate Windsor | Tea | Tea | 0.59 |
| Kokasana | Tea | Tea | 0.46 |
| Harina De Coca | Nutritional Supplement | Ground Leaf | 0.65 |
| Coca Premium | Nutritional Supplement | Ground Leaf | 0.59 |
| Shampoo | Beauty Product | Liquid | N/A |

# Section Six: The Wise & The Foolish

*Now For Some Fun: Angelo Mariani, Master Coca Wine Maker*

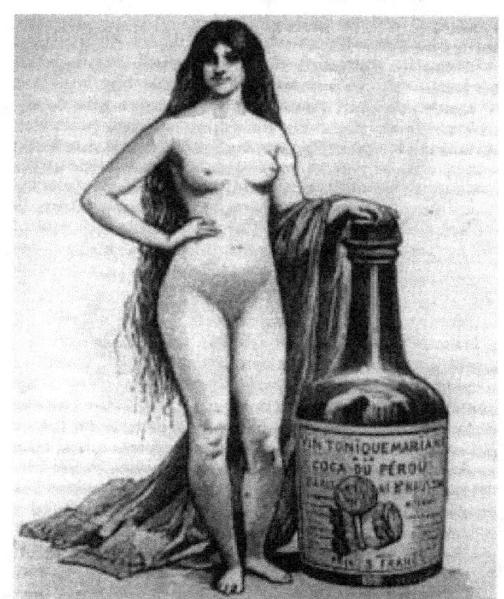

Angelo Mariani was a Corsican/French explorer and innovator who lived in the mid-late 1800's and who, in the course of searching the southern Andes for natural medicines, came across the Coca plant in Bolivia and Peru. By his telling he knew immediately that he had discovered one of nature's true miracle medicines, and he set out to bring it to the world – although it had been in the world of the Andean people for millennia. He spent many years in Bolivia, often returning to France and his greenhouses and production facilities there. He ultimately founded several Coca plantations and production facilities in Bolivia that flourished for many years. He also regularly bought entire Coca harvests from small growers who produced the highest quality leaf.

After years of experimenting with different tonics and elixirs he developed a recipe for producing a healing tonic that he called "Vin Mariani", which as it turned out was a simple extract of pure, whole Coca leaf in high quality Bordeaux red wine. When I say "simple extract" I am understating the tremendous amount of work that Mariani put into the development of his medicine. He made many trips to South America to study the properties of Coca leaf, and ultimately decided that if he was going to be able to control the quality of the leaf he used he would have to grow the Coca himself, and he wound up with three large Coca growing operations in Bolivia and Peru, ensuring that he had a steady supply of the highest quality leaf to ship back to France, where he also made sure that the Bordeaux red wine he was using came from some of the best, most dependable chateaus.

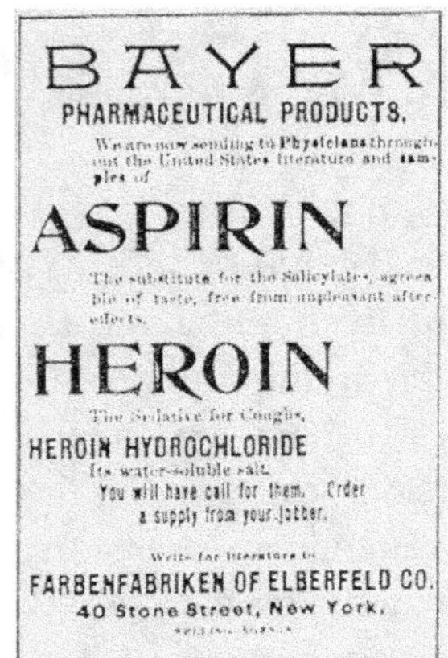


In short, Angelo Mariani was one of the few producers of natural herbal medicines who put in the time, effort and capital to actually make a viable medicine in this era of quacks and con-men whose products were always made with the cheapest ingredients, often containing substances that were know to be toxic, even deadly, but who didn't care because there were always new customers to replace the ones that they addicted and killed.

Not that different than the approach of Pig Pharma today who, if they were not at least somewhat regulated, would be right out there selling snake oil just like their pathological forerunners in the 1800's. And, truly unfortunately, even today there would be millions of desperate people lining up to demand the "miracle cure".

Because Angelo Mariani and his dedication to quality and to producing a medicine that actually helped to cure people of painful, debilitating and deadly conditions, I have compiled and edited (for clarity) one of Mariani's most interesting and useful books "<u>The Therapeutic Applications Of Coca</u>"

### *Of Coca and Its True Therapeutic Properties*

"On chewing Coca leaves one feels a certain dryness of the throat, it produces at the same time a hypersecretion of the salivary glands, and a short while afterward the mucous membrane of the mouth is to a certain extent anesthetized. On its arrival in the stomach, the secretion of the gastric is increased, also the beating of the pulse; the rises about one-half and the urinary secretion is far from diminished."

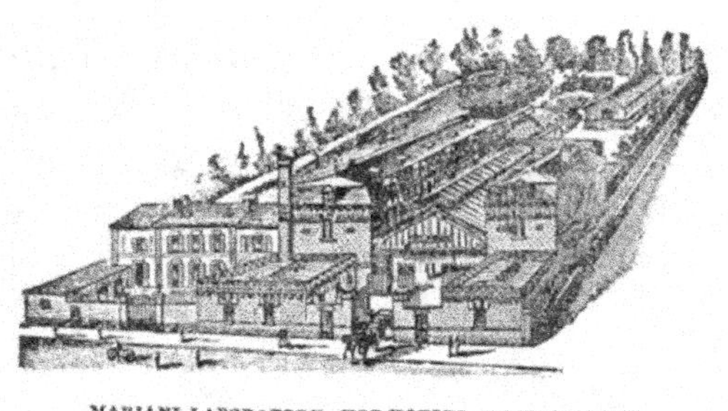

MARIANI LABORATORY, HOT-HOUSES, WINE CELLARS AND WORKSHOPS, NEUILLY-SUR-SEINE, FRANCE.

"Dr. Rabuteau found this in patients afflicted with gout, rheumatism and he has also found under the active influence of Coca, an increase of urea of about 10 per cent took place. Dr. Chas. Fauvel is another one of the first physicians who has experimented clinically with this plant. In a remarkable work, which he published some time ago, Dr. Fauvel praises Coca very highly in affections of the pharynx and of the larynx, and mentions in support of his recommendations several observations of granulous pharyngitis which had resisted all kinds of treatment, but which be had completely cured by the use of Vin Mariani."

"Among all the pharmaceutical of which Coca is the base, we must mention especially the wine prepared by M. Mariani. This skillful chemist has succeeded in so dissolving the active principles of Coca, in a wine that contains already some tannin and traces of iron, that he has made of the whole a tonic "par excellence." This wine is not only agreeable to the taste, but also has the virtue of never constipating; it is, therefore, a thousand times preferable to the different preparations of Cinchona Wine, of which the overrated has fallen considerably since has taken possession of it."

A light and sandy soil, a mean temperature of from fifteen to eighteen and a certain quantity of moisture, are the essential conditions for the perfect growth of Coca. According to Papig, in the valleys of Chincao and Oassapit, the ground where Coca best flourishes is slanting, relatively steep, but very fertile, composed of brick-red clay, containing probably some iron. Coca seeds are sown in beds, called "almazigos."

"The young plants are protected from the heat of the sun's rays by means of straw mats, or woven branches, and are afterward transplanted in furrows about 18 centimetres wide, and 8 deep, about 1 foot apart from each other. Under the beneficial influence of the sun and rain, the growth of the young tree is rapid; it blossoms at the end of from four .to six months, and soon yields seed. The Coca tree attains its complete height (two metres and a half on an average) at the end of about five years."

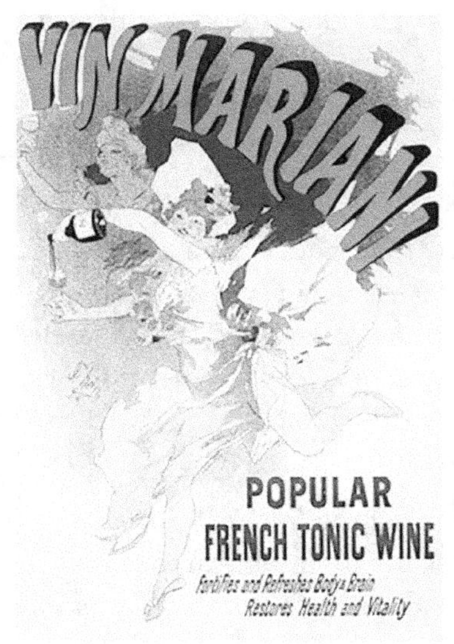



"Attempts have been made to acclimatize it in Europe, but so far without success. Frail specimens may be found in the botanical gardens of and other cities, and also at the establishments of some of the great horticulturists of Belgium. We have given some samples of the plant to the esteemed director of the Jardin Zoologique d'acclimatation of Paris, Mr. Geoffroy Saint-Hilaire, who had them placed in the conservatories of the where the public are admitted to see them. Corsica and Algiers seem to possess the climatic conditions necessary for the perfect development of the Coca, and for that reason it is in these two countries where we shall pursue our efforts of culture."

## *Coca's Known Medical Benefits c. 1880*

"It would not difficult to prolong the list of maladies in which Coca may prove and has proved valuable as a remedy, nor perhaps profitably to discuss its introduction into general use as a substitute for tea and coffee, and especially for chewing tobacco. I will indulge in one remark only.

"That nervousness, many and to a degree before unknown in any country, is being rapidly developed in this land and age, is a melancholy fact to which the American physicians are being speedily opened. Our climate is stimulating, our habits are stimulating, the grounds for existence are stimulating, and human nature is over-driven on every side. May not Coca be destined to the grand palliative of these conditions, and the useful sustainer of exertion among our professional and business men? Contributing so marvelously to endurance both of mind and body, and doing this with certainly less injury to the system than any cognate substance known, I look to Coca as the great preserver of life and health in future generations.

"From what has been said of the nature and effects of Coca it will be seen that I do not regard this plant the light of a drug, any more, at least, than coffee, tea, or tobacco can be so termed. Nor, indeed, is it as susceptible of application as a drug as those substances even; since its effects upon the body are by much disturbance than those of any of them.

"To be of value as a substance must have pathogenetic power. It is, then, not as a drug that we should regard though its sphere in medical practice is destined to be a very wide, and an immensely important one. Its place is that of a food, or, if you supplemental or adjunct to food. Its economic uses in the community will be of a high grade, and employment in the army, navy, merchant marine will be still higher. It will sustain the life of many an exhausted soldier and ship- wrecked sailor.

"Had our army at Gettysburg been supplied with it, Lee and his troops would never have been allowed to re-cross the Potomac. A bale of it should form part of the supply of every ship, since, in case of shipwreck, it would sustain life much longer than a corresponding amount of food. Physiology teaches us that where there is use in the body, there is waste: where there is waste, there must be repair: for repair there must be food; and for food to become fitted repair, there must be digestion and assimilation.

"All this is true, but we must farther, and recall the fact that each mouthful contains a definite, fixed, and practically invariable amount of each element contained in the food. Doubtless the normal proportion of these elements would be the proper one to furnish suitable material for repair in case we were born ·physiologically perfect, and then lived physiologically.' But few of us are born with approach to perfection of structure, and none us can live physiologically.

And this for two reasons:

First: We do not know all of nature's laws

And, second, we could not obey them if we did.

"The demands of life, civilized or savage, prevent it. Probably nature demands that we should go naked. We cannot do it. It demands a proper relation of exercise, food, and sleep. We cannot attain to it; and so on ad infinitum. Now, consider the case of the sedentary man. Does he not waste his brain out of all proportion to his muscles? And is it not clear that to nourish brain, he must eat more muscle-food than he requires? And that at the best must not his brain often go hungry? What becomes of this overplus of muscle-food? Well, two things happen. If the man's stomach is feeble it refuses to digest so much food, and he develops dyspepsia. If he does digest it, and it is absorbed, his blood is filled up with material which he cannot or does not use: his liver becomes congested and, in ordinary parlance, he is bilious.

"Now, are not dyspepsia and biliousness the diseases, par excellence, of sedentary men? And is it not true that literary men, of inactive bodily habit and abstemious as to stimulants, are eaters? If you do not know you have only to ask any housewife who is accustomed to entertain the clergy-a class who avoid wine and tobacco, a part of whom only are able to take tea and coffee in sufficient amount to diminish excessive waste without rendering them nervous; and who are therefore obliged to eat hugely

"For these and all classes in the community upon whom the demands of life are similar, Coca is, in my opinion, infinitely better than wine or tobacco, even with the addition of coffee and tea, and this for reasons already given. Only less important to the laboring classes is it, as bulk of the muscles and other of the body exceeds that of the brain. A surplus of brain food is of small account to the laborer compared with the surplus of food to the sedentary.

"Fat can be stored up in the body or burnt as fuel, and phosphorus, etc., can be easily eliminated by the kidneys. The surplus, being much smaller this instance, can more easily disposed of. Still, he would be a bold man who would say that the laborer is liable to no disease through the lack of a proper relation of food to his exact wants. Now, it can be shown that tea, coffee, wine, tobacco, and, more than all, Coca, prevent waste. And not this alone, but they prevent excess of waste in parts excessively used, or called upon for an undue proportion of work. This way they help to balance up between the needs of the system, under strain of life, the constant and uniform proportion of the elements of food. Who shall measure the benefit of this effect? It is beyond all human computation.

"If, then, my philosophy and physiology be correct, and if Coca is and does what is claimed, and what I believe it will proven to be and do, the introduction of this substance into general use is a matter of exceeding importance, and its employment should be fostered by every true physician.

### *Coca Leaf Wine – Europe's Natural Coca Medicine*
*(Author's note – the following passages are Angelo Mariani speaking, from his book 'The Therapeutic Value of Coca'.)*

"Our Vin Mariani is the first of the preparations of Coca and the one most generally adopted; to the tonic and stimulant action of the drug there is added that of a choice quality of wine. The Vin Coca Mariana contains the soluble parts of the Peruvian plant. The combination of Coca with the tannin and the slightest trace of iron which this wine naturally contains is pronounced to be the most efficacious of tonics. The Coca leaves that we employ after careful selection come from three different sources and are of incomparable quality. It is this that gives to our wine that special taste and agreeable aroma which renders it so acceptable to the sick."

"It is likewise to the combination of these three varieties of Coca leaf in our wine that we can attribute this important fact: during almost 30 years, no matter in how large doses taken, Vin Mariani has never produced cocainism.  (We caution especially against the many so-called Coca wines made with the alkaloid Cocaine alone.)"

"Vin Mariani is a diffusable tonic, the action of which is immediate. This action, instead of being localized on a single organ, the stomach, spreads to the whole system. Taken into the circulation, it awakens in its course the retarded functions of every organ, and this is owing to the presence in our preparation of the volatile principles of the plant."

"Unlike other tonics, the astringent properties of which lead at length to heat and constipation, Vin Mariani does not produce any disorder of the digestive functions; it stimulates them, exerts a refreshing action on the gastric mucous membrane, and on that account so advantageously replaces the preparations of cinchona, iron, strychnine, etc."

"There is," says Dr. Mallez, "a form of anæmia to which the attention of physicians has not yet been called, and which yields marvelously to the employment of Vin Mariani; we allude to that state of profound depression of the economy, of extremely marked impoverishment of the blood, which also results from the prolonged abuse of balsamics in the treatment of diseases of the urinary passages."

"The number of persons who, attacked with blennorrhagia, use cubebs, copaiba, turpentine, etc., to a deplorable extent is considerable. So true is this that, out of a hundred young dyspeptics, we may affirm without fear of being in error that at least forty of them have become so by the use of balsamics."

{Gazette cies Hopitciux, Nov.  23, 1877.)

## *Mariani's Medicinal Coca Leaf Preparations*

### Coca Leaf Tea

*Take of Coca leaves, bruised, one ounce; boiling water ten fluid ounces. (Editor's Note — using pure water heated to 180o F at sea level yields a better tea.) Infuse in a covered vessel for one hour, press slightly, strain; there will be obtained a fluid measuring about eight ounces, having an appearance and odour like unto an infusion of ordinary green tea. (Editor's note: the use of a widely available coffee brewing device called a "French Press" is an ideal tea brewing/pressing vessel.) Slightly alkaline and bitter in taste. Dose, from half to one and a half fluid ounces, each fluid ounce representing one dram of leaves.*

### Aqueous Extract of Coca Leaf

*Coca leaves, bruised, or, what is better, in coarse powder, eight ounces, water a sufficiency. Macerate the coca in two pints of water, at a temperature of 120° F., for a period of two hours. Pack in a conical percolator, and exhaust with water at a temperature of 100° F. Evaporate by water bath, at a temperature not exceeding 140° F., to the required consistence. This extract is brownish in colour, and bitter in taste. Dose, ten to twenty-five grains.*

### Alcohol Extract of Coca Leaf

*Coca in moderately coarse powder; alcohol, 56 over proof, a sufficiency. Moisten the powder with alcohol; pack in a conical percolator. Add more alcohol and continue the percolation until the powder is exhausted. Evaporate the resulting percolate, by means of a water bath at a temperature not exceeding 140o F., until of a proper consistence for forming pills. This is much superior to the aqueous extract, possessing the characteristic taste and odour of coca-leaves in a high degree. It is of a green colour, resinous or waxy in character, due to the presence of coca-wax. Dose, five to fifteen grains in the form of pills. (Mariani's lozenges with the addition of flavorings such as mint or licorice were produced using this formulation method.)*

### Fluid Extract of Coca Leaf

*Coca in coarse powder, eight ounces, proof spirit, a sufficiency. Moisten the leaves with proof spirit, pack tightly in a percolator, pour on proof spirit, until six ounces of percolate has been obtained which set aside; then exhaust the leaves with more proof spirit, evaporate, at a temperature of 140° F., to a bulk of two ounces, which add to the first percolate. Dose, forty-five to ninety minims.*

### Glycerin Extract of Coca Leaf

*Take Coca leaves, in coarse powder, five ounces; on which pour two ounces of hot water, then add fifteen ounces (by weight) of glycerin. Macerate, in a warm place, for a period of thirty days. At the end of that time press out the fluid portion, using a screw press, strain the resulting fluid product and set aside. Remove the residue from the press, and pour on it about twenty-four ounces of water at a temperature of 150° F., at which temperature let it be kept for a period of two hours; strain, evaporate to such a product that the quantity when added to the glycerin fluid shall measure fifteen fluid ounces. This is a very pleasant and efficient preparation of Erythroxylon coca and is generally admissable in all cases. Dose, one to three drams.*

### Tincture of Coca Leaf

*Coca leaves, bruised or in coarse powder, four ounces; proof spirit, one pint. Moisten the leaves, pack in a percolator, and percolate twenty ounces. Dose, four, to six or eight drams. This form is very objectionable, as the amount of alcohol administered in a dose of the tincture will altogether alter the natural effects of the coca-leaf.*

### Mama Coca & The Exploiters

A widespread patent medicine trade developed in the US in the mid-late 1800's with the emerging awareness of the power of Coca Leaf as a natural medicine. The developers of these tonics ranged from sincere physicians to fraudulent opportunists, and the most effective tonics were those made from real Coca leaf with no added toxic or addictive ingredients. ingredients. One of the most popular was a simple extract of Coca Leaf called "Coca Cordial" by a young American company that was becoming a big player in patent medicines of all kinds, which evolved into the industry I believe it's fair to refer to as Pig Pharma today.

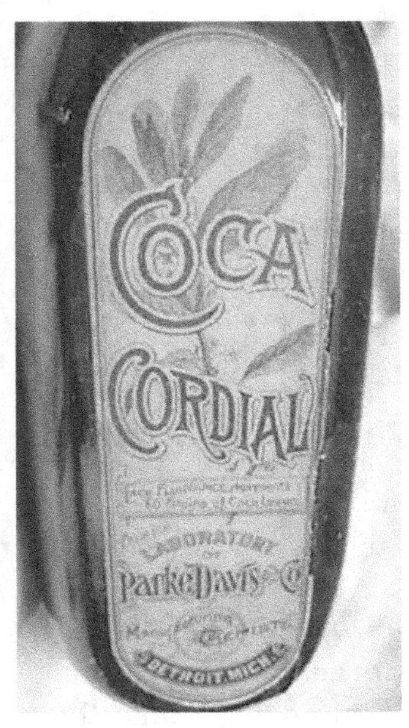


Parke, Davis & Company distributed millions of bottles of Coca Cordial advertised heavily as a "Palatable Preparation of Coca Erythroxylon Containing in an agreeable vehicle the active medicinal principle, free from the bitter astringent constituents of the drug."

The American "Tonic trade" targeted women heavily, and Coca Cordial was pitched as being prepared especially for "persons of delicate nervous organization". This 1880's tonic, one of hundreds, was recommended for treating nervous exhaustion, irritability, indigestion, depression, nausea, vomiting, alcoholism, or opium abuse. It was said to have a "rich vinous flavor", probably because "each fluid ounce contains 60 grains of coca leaves" offering an amazing range of "sedative, tonic, and stimulant effects." It would be interesting to see this exact product back on the market today, wouldn't it? However, there was a catch in the 1880's:

> *"The widespread distribution of cocaine in cola beverages and in popular remedies such as "Coca Cordial" meant that American physicians and dentists had little explaining to do when offering patients cocaine as a local anesthetic." (American Society of Anesthesiologists)*

### Identifying & Extracting The Magic Bullet

Like far too many aspects of modern life the production of Cocaine has gotten cruder, and more toxic over the years. For a detailed look at the crude, toxic methods and materials used by the drug cartels in producing the Cocaine that sells on the streets of the US and Europe, check out these US government-sponsored fully-illustrated directions for how to manufacture Cocaine in the jungle: *https://tinyurl.com/n7fh4aw* Assuming the link is still live, that's a DEA website with full instructions on how the bad guys make Cocaine. DEA likes to show off and mock the primitive methods used by the cartels. As if they aren't knuckle-draggers themselves.

The world of Mama Coca wasn't always this way. Today's Cocaine bears only a chemical resemblance to the Cocaine that was being produced in the 1800's by pharmacy labs and even by doctors themselves for their patients.

Enlightened early chemical explorers focused on the Cocaine alkaloid as only one part of a synergistic whole, even while working to extract and understand its miraculous properties:

*"The wholly different action of cocaine therapeutically from the Coca leaves of the Andean, or the more exact scientific preservations of Coca such as exhibited in the preparations of M. Mariani - which fully represents the action of recent Peruvian Coca, clearly indicates the presence of certain important principles in Coca, the properties of which are sufficiently distinct to markedly effect physiological action in a manner different from any one of its alkaloids. Happily we are now learning more definitely through research and experimentation, and these earlier errors are being corrected."*

### *Search For The Secrets Of The Coca Leaf*

"Of all the problems in the study of Coca the search for the force producing qualities of the leaf is the most profound. Science, ever alert to trace with exactitude the secrets of Nature, has struggled in vain to isolate and explain this hidden source of energy. But so cleverly are the atoms associated which go to build up the molecules of power in this marvelous leaf, that though the chemist through the delicacy of analysis has from time to time placed these atoms in differing groups and thus often given to the world some new combination, the one sought element of pent-up endurance inherent in Coca has remained concealed. It is like the secret of life - though known to be broadly dependent on certain principles which may readily be explained, the knowledge of the one essential element remains as great a secret as before research began.

"Though all the accounts of travelers had directed attention to the peculiar qualities of Coca in sustaining strength, at the period when the first knowledge of this leaf reached Europe chemistry was not sufficiently advanced to admit of an exact analysis of plant life. Indeed, science met with little encouragement when the great powers were engrossed in political preferment, and it was not until the latter part of the eighteenth century that an impetus seemed given to research after Lavoisier had laid the foundation for modern chemistry. Though he lost his life on the guillotine through the whirligig of political fate during the French

Revolution, just as he was at the height of his labors, a new interest was established and the work of the French chemists became active.

"Humboldt was then making his extensive explorations through South America, collecting data which was to serve as a basis of research during many subsequent years. Cuvier, the anatomist, was advancing his theories on the classification of animals; Fraunhofer had established a means for studying the heavenly bodies through the spectrum, while chemical electricity had progressed from the experiments of Volta to the electromagnet of Ampere.

"The method for expressing chemical equations, such as are now shown by those symbolic letters and figures which appear to the uninitiated as so many hieroglyphics, was not understood until Dalton, in 1808, had perfected his law of proportions. This was an important advance in chemical knowledge, for from it was built up the sign language which in a chemical formula expresses not only the symbol of each element, but tells the chemist the relative proportion of the combining atoms.

> *"These fundamental facts are of interest as bearing upon the chemical history of the Coca leaf, while the combining nature of atoms has suggested an interesting theory that the physiological action of a chemical medicine is influenced by its molecular weight. This has been a matter of discussion among physiological chemists for years, and was suggested by Blake as long ago as 1841 and since by Rabuteau. Thus an element of a fixed atomic weight may have special reference to the muscular system, while another of different weight may act upon the nervous tissue - qualities which are fulfilled in the action of the several Coca bases."*

"It was but a natural outcome of this spirit for research that turned the attention of explorers to South America, which had remained practically a new world since its discovery. Here were to be found innumerable strange plants indigenous to a country where everything was marvelous when viewed with the comparative light of the older world. In the height of this interest, the suggestive hints of naturalists and travelers were incentives to further the investigations of the European chemists. The writings of Cieza, Monardes, Acosta, Garcilasso and a host of others upon the wonderful qualities of the Coca leaf, stimulated a desire to solve its tradition of ages and prove its qualities by the test of science.

> *It is surprising to now look back over three centuries and recall these early authors, to consider under what conditions they wrote, and to read with what enthusiasm and exactness they gave expression to the knowledge they had gained from an observation of the novel customs about them. Thus the Jesuit father, Blas Valera, speaking of the hidden energy of*

*Coca, wrote: "It may be gathered how powerful the Cuca is in its effect on the laborer, from the fact that the Indians who use it become stronger and much more satisfied and work all day without eating."*

### The Curious Necessity Of Lipita

"Attention was very naturally directed to the method in which Coca was used, and the llipta (note: this is 'lime', or calcium carbonate) which was employed with the leaves in chewing was looked upon as having some decided influence. Dr. Unanue, who has written much concerning the customs of the Indians, was one of the first to suggest that possibly this alkaline addition to the leaf developed some new property to which the qualities of Coca might be attributed, while Humboldt, as elsewhere referred to, through an error of observation considered this added lime as the supposed property of endurance."

"Stevenson, in 1825, described the action of the llipta as altering the insipid taste of the leaves so as to render them sweet, and in 1827 Poeppig expressed the opinion that there was a volatile constituent in the Coca leaf which exposure to the air completely destroys."

### Attention Turns To Alkaloids

Attention had now been directed to the isolation of alkaloids from plants, and during the first quarter of the nineteenth century several active principles were thus obtained and the possibility of tracing the hidden properties of Coca through analysis was suggested. Von Tschudi, when engaged in his extended explorations through Peru, became so impressed with the qualities of Coca that he advised Mr. Pizzi, Director of the Laboratory Botica y Drogueria Boliviana at La Paz, to examine the leaves, which resulted in the discovery of a supposed alkaloid, but when on his return to Germany this body was shown to Woehler, it was found to be merely plaster of Paris, the result of some careless manipulation.

Dr. Weddell, in 1850, after a prolonged personal experience in the Andes with the sustaining effects of Coca, pronounced it as yielding a stimulant action differing from that of all other excitants. This influence both he and other observers supposed might be due to the presence of theine, the active principle of tea, which had shortly before been discovered, and was then exciting considerable discussion. With this idea in view, Coca leaves were examined, and, though this substance was not found, there was obtained a peculiar body, soluble in alcohol, insoluble in ether, very bitter, and incapable of crystallization, and a tannin was obtained to which was attributed the virtues of Coca.

About this same period there was found in the leaves a peculiar volatile resinous matter of powerful odor, and two years later, from a distillation of the dry residue of an aqueous extract of Coca, an oily liquor of a smoky odor was separated together with a sublimate of small needle-like crystals, which was named "Erythroxyline," after the family of which Coca is a species.

### *Where The "Magic Bullet" Hunters Went Astray*

*(Author's note — throughout the following sections you'll find the works of a lot of writers referred to; there are links in the bibliography to the digitized works of all the writers referenced anywhere in the book.)*

'The wholly different action of cocaine therapeutically from the Coca leaves of the Andean, or the more exact scientific preservations of Coca such as exhibited in the preparations of M. Mariani - which fully represents the action of recent Peruvian Coca, clearly indicates the presence of certain important principles in Coca, the properties of which are sufficiently distinct to markedly effect physiological action in a manner different from any one of its alkaloids. Happily we are now learning more definitely through research and experimentation, and these earlier errors are being corrected.

"The diametrically opposite findings of investigators of known repute indicate that these inharmonious conclusions were not wholly the result of carelessness nor prejudice. Just as Coca experimented with by one observer repeated the traditional influence, or in some other instance proved inert, so the chemists found the result of their labors at variance. Much of this confusion was cleared away when the botanists explained that there are several varieties of Coca. Those qualities which had formerly been attributed to superstitious belief, or which when reluctantly accepted as possibly present in an extremely fugitive form which was lost through volatility, were shown to be dependent upon the variety as much as upon the quality of the Coca leaf employed in the process of manufacture.

"Cocamine, $C_{19}H_{23}NO_4$, (*author's note – this is Cocaine*) was originally studied in the alkaloids obtained from the small leaf variety of Coca by Hesse. It was regarded by Liebermann as identical with a base which he described as y-isatropyl-cocaine and afterward termed a truxilline, because supposedly found only in the Truxillo variety of Coca.

"The research leading to these conclusions provoked bitter controversy between these two investigators. It has since been determined that cocamine is of the same empirical composition as cocaine, though weaker in anaesthetic action. It is a natural product of several varieties of Coca, particularly of that grown in Java. From hydrolysis by mineral acids cocamine yields cocaic, iso-cocaic and homo-iso-cocaic acids, while from its isomeride there is formed in a similar way alpha-isotropic or beta-truxillic acid. Both cocaic and iso-cocaic acids yield cinnamic acid and other products on distillation. Subsequently a similar body was prepared synthetically from ecgonine and cinnamic anhydride, and named cinnamyl-cocaine. It forms large colorless crystals, melts at 1200, is almost insoluble in water, and readily soluble in alcohol and ether. This body has been proved to occur naturally in Coca leaves from various sources, being present in some specimens as high as 0.5 per cent.

"Thus it will be seen there has been much discussion and uncertainty upon the Coca products, particularly so as to those of an oily nature, originally designated as hygrine and the amorphous substances previously described under various titles.

"It is the opinion of Hesse that hygrine is a product of decomposition of one of the Coca bases, and does not occur in fresh Coca leaves; in support of which he asserted that while dilute acid solutions of hygrine have a strongly marked blue florescence which is characteristic, this reaction is not shown when fresh leaves are first operated upon. But as this reaction develops gradually, he inferred that hygrine was formed by the decomposition of amorphous cocaine, from the solution of which it could be separated by ammonia and caustic soda as a colorless oil having the odor of quinoline. In fact, he considered the oil thus obtained a homologue of quinoline, possibly a tri-methyl-quinoline.

"Another observer, while experimenting with the alkaloids of Coca by means of their platinum salts, obtained an oily base, exceedingly bitter and differing in odor and solubility from that which had been described by Lessen, but which was presumably identical with the amorphous products, cocaicine and cocainiodine, and Hesse concluded there might really be two oily bases in amorphous cocaine, one found in the benzoyl compounds of the broad leaf variety and one in the cinnamyl compounds of the Novo Granatense variety, in both cases associated with cocamine and another base, which he named cocrylamine. Liebermann, on the other hand, considers hygrine a combination of two liquid oxygenated bases which may be separated by fractional distillation. One - $C_8H_{15}NO$, an isomeride of tropine, with a boiling point 1930 to 195°, the other, $C_{14}H_{24}N_2O$, not distilling under ordinary pressure without decomposition, while still other experimenters from distilling barium ecgonate obtained a volatile oily liquid which strongly resembles hygrine. Merck has shown this body yields, on decomposition, methylamine, from which it has been inferred that it is identical with tropine, and hence closely allied to atropine. With this fact in view it was presumed the dilating property of cocaine upon the pupil was due to hygrine, but this has been proved not to be the case.

### What Happened To The Cocaine?

The assertion that hygrine is never present in Coca leaves, but is merely a decomposition product in the manufacture of cocaine, lends an added interest to the research of Dr. Kusby upon fresh Coca leaves made while he was at Bolivia. From repeated examinations he found a certain yield of alkaloids, while specimens of the same leaves sent to the United States yielded from treatment by the same process less than half the percentage of alkaloid that he had obtained. This prompted him to search for the possible source of error, and it was found that after all the cocaine was eliminated there was still a decided alkaloidal precipitate. From this it was concluded that: "native Coca leaves contain a body intimately associated with the cocaine and reacting to the same test, which almost wholly disappears from them in transit."

This result indicates the presence in Coca leaves of some extremely volatile principle to which decided physiological properties are attached, which may also be obtained from suitably preserved leaves. When a preparation made from recent leaves in Bolivia was submitted to Professor Remsen, of Johns Hopkins University, his assistant reported that he found a bitter principle, and an oil, which presumably differed in no way from that found at the time of the examinations made in Bolivia. This is comparable with similar findings of those who have experimented with Coca, whether the leaves were recent and examined on the spot, or the examination had been made thousands of miles distant upon well preserved leaves. In each instance similar volatile alkaloids have been obtained, which have commonly been pronounced "decomposition products," yet, as these are always found by careful observers, it indicates they are the natural associate bases of Coca.

## Appendix One – A Physician's Testimony

*(Author's note: I'm including this well-written and thoroughly-researched report by a widely-respected 19th Century physician on both his research and his personal experiences with Coca, which he terms Cuca, as well as his reporting of the findings of other physicians of his time. It's easy to see why Pig Pharma doesn't want people to be able to grow their own Coca Leaf as easily as they can grow Basil and Parsley, or Cannabis for that matter in their home gardens. Also note that you can access all of the writers the author refers to in the bibliography of this book.)*

**"Observations On The Effects Of Cuca, Or Coca, The Leaves Of Erythroxylon Coca".** By Sir Robert Christison, Bart., M.D., (in) British Medical Journal, April 29, 1876

'THE brief notice taken in my introductory address to this Society in November last, of the restorative and preservative virtues of the Peruvian Cuca or coca-leaf against bodily fatigue from severe exercise, has led to numberless references to me by friends and strangers in all parts of the kingdom for information as to its effects, its safety, its applicability to the treatment of some states of disease, and the quarters in which it may be obtained.

## Background On Coca, Or Cuca

'As I am not aware of any trials of it having been made in this country, either earlier than mine or so extensive, and as I shall probably best answer the many inquiries sent me by publishing an account of these experiments, I have been induced to present the following narrative to the Botanical Society. The inquiry, of which my recent trials form a part, is very far from being complete, because my supply was quite inadequate till the other day, when I received a sufficiency through the kind services of my colleague Professor Wyville Thomson, of the Challenger expedition.

"But the facts already obtained will probably interest not a few at the present time, were it for no more than that they set at rest all doubts that the more important of the effects of Cuca, experienced in its own country by the natives of Peru and the neighbouring states, may be equally produced in Europeans at home; and that, contrary to what seems universally believed in Peru, the virtues of the leaf may be preserved, with due care, for many years.

"Since my observations must bear reference to what is the doctrine and practice of the Peruvians as to the use of this vegetable, I must introduce the subject with a summary of what has been written about it by the historians of Peru and by travellers in that country. The accounts which have thus appeared—from time to time are apparently very contradictory; but I think they may be reconciled, and a consistent result obtained.

"In the first place, however, let me remark that I have ventured to restore to the commercial article its original name, Cuca. This was Its Indian name, which the Spaniards corrupted into coca. But there is no reason why other nations should adopt a Spanish corruption; and there is a very good argument against transferring it to our own tongue, inasmuch as we have already two totally different vegetable products, cocoa and cacao, which, as indiscriminately pronounced in ordinary speech, coco and coca, are undistinguishable from the corrupt name of this new invention. I hope, therefore, that others will second me in attaching a characteristic name to an article which seems very likely to come ere long into general use among our countrymen at home.

"The early historians of Peru have taken special notice of the culture, properties, and uses of Cuca. Among these, none is more full, clear, and fair, than the famous chronicler of the reign of the Incas and of the Spanish conquest, Garcilasso de la Vega. His narrative bears internal evidence of great historical care. Other reasons, to be alluded to presently, also add to the confidence which the statements themselves create in the reader; and hence it is scarcely necessary to refer to any other early authority. Garcilasso's information was derived partly from what he personally knew, partly from a Spanish priest, Blas Valera, who was long in Peru, and whose manuscripts came into the historian's possession.

"De la Vega informs us that the use of Cuca in Peru dates from an early period of the dominion of the Incas; that at first it was scarce, and was monopolised by the monarchs themselves; that it was employed as an offering to the sun, their parent and deity; and that sometimes, however, a basket of it was presented to one of their curacas, or lords, to whom the ruler desired to show special favour. But, as the Incas extended their conquests northward along the Cordilleras of the Andes, the culture of the plant also became much more widely extended, through the acquisition of suitable lands for the purpose; the leaves came gradually into more general use; and at the time of the Spanish conquest of Peru, the natives almost universally indulged in Cuca-chewing.

### The Attackers Encircle Mama Coca

"The Spaniards, however, were too devoted Catholics to fall into a custom which was the offspring, and continued to have the savour, of profane heathen rites. The chewing of Cuca was detested by them, condemned by public opinion, and charged with being baneful to the health of those who gave themselves up to it. Strong prejudices thus prevailed against it. But Garcilasso de la Vega and Blas Valera protest against these prejudices, and declare that the Peruvian natives esteemed Cuca as above gold and silver in value; that it possessed great energy in preserving strength during fatiguing exercise and privation of food; that it was an useful medicine for improving the teeth, mending broken bones, curing maggoty sores, and warding off the effects of cold; and that another important purpose served by it was to enrich the Spanish traders in it, and to supply the chief tithes of the cathedral and canons of Cuzco.

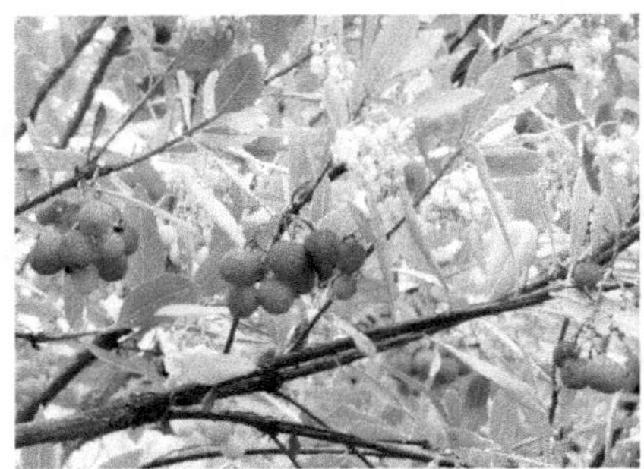

"The plant is described as a shrub about six feet high, much resembling in foliage the strawberry-tree of Spain (Arbutus Unedo - left), but producing much thinner leaves; and it is stated that the gatherers pick off the leaves individually with caution; dry them quickly in the sun, so as to retain their green colour, which is much prized; and preserve them carefully from damp, which seriously damages their quality. Garcilasso adds an anecdote which illustrates both the Spanish dislike and the real virtues of Cuca.

*A Spanish friend of his met one of his countrymen, a poor soldier, plodding his solitary way among the Andes, chewing Cuca, and carrying his two-year-old child in his arms. On upbraiding the man for adopting a barbarian custom, abhorred by all true believers as the fruit and symbol of idolatrous worship, the soldier said that might be; he at one time shared in these prejudices, but had found he could not carry his child without the strength which the Cuca imparted, and was too poor to afford the cost of a bearer to relieve him of his burden. Nowhere does the author of the Royal Commentaries of the Incas say one word of any evil consequences actually resulting from the use of this vegetable becoming a habit.*

"In face of the opposition it received from subsequent authors, and from some modern travellers, this testimony of Garcilasso de la Vega may be received with favour. He was son of one of Pizarro's conquering captains of the same name, by a niece of one of the last of the Incas. He would, therefore, escape the tendency of the pure Spanish race to vilify the manners and customs of the people they had subdued; and his native and royal extraction gave him access to full information on such a subject. It is true that he left the land of his birth at the age of twenty (in 1550), and passed the remainder of a long life in Spain. But a youth of his family extraction on both sides was old enough to take part in the stirring events of the period while he remained at Cuzco; and, after leaving it for Spain, he kept up correspondence with the friends he left behind him, collecting from them information for his history.

"I was first led to pay attention to the Peruvian custom of chewing Cuca by reading, full forty years ago, the Travels in Chilé, Peru, and on the River Amazons, of the German naturalist Pöppig, who has taken a very different view of this national custom from Garcilasso de la Vega and Blas Valera.

"Pöppig was no less than five years in these regions, from 1827 to 1832, and passed much of his time among the Cuca-chewers in the forest regions of the Peruvian Andes. Probably no European in the present century had such opportunities of intimately studying the habit. His statements of fact and his opinions are, therefore, entitled to much consideration.

*"The conclusion at which he arrived is that "The habit is as seductive and as injurious to health, mind, and morals as that of tippling in Europe, or opium-eating in the East. He says it is almost confined to natives of the aboriginal red race, has not been adopted by negroes, and is discountenanced among all of European descent; that even those who use it to no great excess must stop their work several times a-day to chew their quid contemplatively, and are much displeased if disturbed in their placid enjoyment; and that those who have got thus far are apt to become mere slaves to it, surrender every other occupation for it, and, quitting society, pass their time in the wild forests between hunting for their sustenance and lying under a tree chewing their beloved weed, calling up delightful visions and building castles in the air, and so insensible to outward occurrences as to remain thus all night indifferent to cold, torrents of rain, and even the howlings of the panther in their neighbourhood."*

*"But, in the end, the stomach gives way; the countenance becomes haggard, and the limbs emaciated; they can no longer take sufficient food, and even lose all relish for the enjoyment which has been insidiously destroying them; constipation sets in, even obstruction of the bowels ensues, or jaundice, or dropsy; and thus at last life is cut short about the age of fifty by one or other of these maladies, or through simple extenuation and exhaustion. Sometimes, when a fit of excess is followed by dislike, and the habit is suddenly abandoned, the sufferer rallies, and seems about to be reclaimed. But, ere long, like the drink-craver in exactly the same circumstances, he is driven by an uncontrollable impulse to further and worse indulgence."*

*"When the habit has thus degenerated into a vice, the victim becomes, in the language of the country, a Coquero, and is irreclaimable. If a man of Spanish blood begin to use Cuca, he is at once looked on with suspicion; for usually, in the course of time, he abandons himself entirely to it, and becomes an outcast from the society in which he moved."*

"Pöppig gives, among other instances, a melancholy tale of a young man of good station in Huanuco, who fell into this vice, lived for some time the life of a savage. in the woods, was found out by his relatives in a miserable condition in a remote native village, and was brought back to town by force, and for a short time apparently reclaimed. But at length, eluding his friends, he fled back again to the mountains, and resumed the habits of a confirmed Coquero.

"It is unnecessary to follow Pöppig further through the arguments and illustrations, very interesting however, by which he was led to denounce Cuca as a deceitful and destructive stimulant of the narcotic kind.

He allows, nevertheless, that it has really wonderful power in supporting the strength under prolonged fatigue without food. He mentions that, in his long rides through the Peruvian forests, he had seen his Indian followers accompany him on foot for fifty miles in one day, without food, or anything else except Cuca; and that, in the revolutionary wars which ended with the Spanish American States throwing off subjection to old Spain, the native Peruvian troops, poorly clothed and ill fed, were able to fall upon their enemies by surprise, by making long marches among the mountains without food or sleep, merely resting for intervals of a few minutes occasionally to refresh themselves by Cuca chewing.

"He adds an important fact, which I am able to confirm, that, when his day's journey came to an end, he did not find his Indian attendants had at all lost their appetites; for, when done with work for the day, although they did not care for food while travelling and chewing, they made an excellent meal in the evening, usually eating twice as much as satisfied his own hunger. These last rather inviting statements will prepare the way for the more favourable testimony of ulterior travellers on the same subject.

## *Reality Trumps Prejudice & Dogma*

"Three valuable observers, who have since spent some time as naturalists in Peru and became familiar with the fondness of the natives for the Cuca-leaf, have treated the question minutely; and they separately bear witness to the soundness of the views of Garcilasso de la Vega and Blas Valera, and to some mistake on the part of Pöppig, for which it is not easy to account. It is important to see to what their testimony exactly amounts. It is by no means sufficient, as some have thought, to set aside Pöppig 's statements, by referring to the wide dissemination of the Peruvian habit. It has been said, indeed, to be nearly universal among a population of eight million inhabiting the Andes; and the annual collection of the leaf has been estimated at no less than thirty millions of pounds. Witt the habit of intoxication with opium, or with alcoholic spirits, might be upheld on the very same plea.

"In 1838, Von Tschudi visited Peru, and was for some time in the neighbourhood of Lima, as well as in various other districts, where the natives of Indian race almost universally use Cuca, and where he himself repeatedly made trial of it.

"Dr. Veddell of Poitiers, who had previously investigated with singular success in Upper Peru the botany of the cinchonas, and was the first to discover there the true yellow bark tree, the most valuable of them all, revisited Bolivia in 1851, where, in the province of Yungas, the finest Cuca is said to be cultivated. He, too, made trial of it himself, and had very ample opportunities of witnessing its use and its effects among the Peruvians.

"In 1860, Clements Markham, who had charge of the Government expeditions to Peru in quest of cinchona plants for cultivation in India, was much in the wildest forest districts of Lower Peru, immediately adjoining Bolivia, was always attended by Cuca-chewing natives, and not unfrequently followed their example.

> *All these authorities, undeniably of the first rank, agree that the repulsive accounts of Pöppig are much exaggerated. The general result of their experience is to raise a suspicion that, in a few instances, his deplorable history of the abandoned irreclaimable Coquero may be not far from the truth. But they do not seem to have themselves met with any such cases.*

"Von Tschudi, indeed, says, that a profligate Coquero may be known by his foul breath, stumpy teeth, pale quivering lips, black-cornered mouth, dim eyes, yellow skin, unsteady gait, and general apathy; but in his narrative, obviously in part compiled, he does not say he described such a man from actual observation; on the contrary, all three travellers represent in colours more or less strong the great utility of Cuca to the Indians in the hard labour they have to undergo.

"Von Tschudi observes that, in his own trials, he found it to be a preventive of that difficulty in breathing which is felt in the rapid ascent of the Andes; that, when frequenting the Peruvian Puna, or great desert table-land, 14,000 feet above the level of the sea, a decoction of the leaves enabled him to climb heights, and pursue swift-footed game, with no greater difficulty than in similar rapid exercise on the coast ; and that he experienced a sense of satiety which did not leave him till the time of the next meal after that which he ought otherwise to have taken. He mentions the following instance, which he carefully watched, of the power of the Indians to bear long fatigue without any other sustenance.

"A miner, sixty-two years old, worked for him at laborious digging five days and nights without food, or more than two hours of sleep nightly, his only support being half an ounce of Cuca leaves every three hours. The man then accompanied him on foot during a ride of sixty miles in two days; and, at parting, expressed himself ready to engage to undertake as much as he had performed. Nevertheless, von Tschudi was assured by the priest of the district that he had never known the man to be ill.

"In general terms, this traveller declares he is clearly of opinion that the moderate use of Cuca not only is innocuous, but may even be conducive to health and, again he observes,"… after long and attentive observation, I am convinced that its use in moderation is nowise detrimental, and that without it the poorly fed Peruvian Indian would be incapable of going through his usual labour. The Cuca plant must be considered a great blessing to Peru"

"Weddell, in less glowing terms, says, that careful inquiry where Cuca is most in use satisfied him that it might be injurious to Europeans not gradually accustomed to it; but that it has the power of sustaining the strength for a time without food, yet without interfering with the appetite soon afterwards; that, in his own trials, he experienced a slight excitement and a little subsequent sleeplessness, but nothing else; and that, in the countries he visited, he never saw things go the length described by Pöppig, who must have been misled by exceptional cases

"The testimony of Clements Markham is very explicit. He says the properties of Cuca are to enable a greater amount of fatigue to be borne with less nourishment and to prevent difficult breathing in the ascent of steep mountain-sides; that, although when used to excess it is prejudicial to the health, yet " … of all the narcotics used by man, it is the least injurious and most soothing and invigorating" ; that he chewed it frequently, and, besides an agreeable soothing feeling, found he could endure long abstinence from food with less inconvenience than he could otherwise have felt; and that it enabled him to ascend precipitous mountain-sides with a feeling of lightness and elasticity, and without losing breath. " It enabled him to ascend the mighty passes of the Andes "… with ease and comfort."

"It is difficult to reconcile with these favourable opinions the very opposite conclusions of Pöppig, founded apparently on personal observation. Probably, he was too prepossessed with the abhorrence with which the practice of chewing Cuca was regarded by the white inhabitants of the towns; hence he might have mistaken for the effects of the habit what perhaps was no more than the physical expression of the natural indolence of the Indian race when indulged in to excess; or, in other cases, the result of over-indulgence in ardent spirits, which, he says, the Coquero sometimes adds to his other vices.

"Mr. Bates met with this habit among the natives on the banks or the river Amazons, where he says it is regarded with abhorrence by respectable people, and therefore only practised secretly. He represents Cuca, there called ypaaå, as stimulating and not injurious when used in moderation, but producing weakness and nervous exhaustion when indulged in to excess. His observations, however, are too brief and general to throw much light on the subject.

### *Detailed Notes On Coca Botany, Cultivation & Treatment*

*The shrub which produces Cuca thrives best in the clearances in the elevated forests of the Andes, in a climate distinguished by frequent rain-showers, and exemption equally from frosts and from extreme heats. In due season it is covered with clusters (fascicles) of delicate white flowers, which give it the appearance of our blackthorn in spring; and the flowers are succeeded by red berries. The plants bear stripping of their leaves three times in the course of the year. Great care is usually taken to nip them off without hurting the axillary buds. They are dried at once quickly and thoroughly, and so as not to curl; at least, all good specimens I have seen present the leaves flattened and many of them entire, almost as if intended as a herbarium.*

*Great care is taken to keep them afterwards dry, when transported from place to place. When newly dried, they have a strong odour, which is said to be apt to cause headache in those frequent the drying-floors for the first time; but this odour passes off by the time the leaves are packed. The packages when opened have a powerful tea-like odour; which they retain on reaching Europe, if duly protected from damp. In Peru it is alleged that their properties soon deteriorate, that in a few months they lose much of their virtue, and that when taken to the coast they are worthless in twelve months. This statement, however, must be received with some limitation.*

*It is evident, from the pains taken in Peru to preserve them from damp and exposure, that the leaves are easily damaged without due precaution; so that neglect will account for the inferiority of many old samples. Besides, it is contrary to all analogy, that leaves destitute of volatile oil, at least not owing their virtue to volatile oil, should lose them under careful preservation from the ordinary causes of decay;*

*and various medicinal leaves of European growth, formerly thought to become inert by keeping, are now, known to retain their properties very long, since we have been aware of the precautions for preserving them. Further, specimens brought to Europe have been found to yield a crystalline principle, which physiologically possesses no mean activity as a narcotic, which is probably the active ingredient, and which apparently bears transport and long keeping well. Lastly, well preserved Cuca will produce in Europe in no small degree, after being kept several years, the remarkable effects on man which are every day experienced in Peru.*

"Cuca is not yet a regular commercial article in this country. In the prospect of its soon becoming so, the characters of a good sample should be well understood. I have had two fine specimens of it, and have seen several evidently much inferior. The fine qualities consist of leaves in a great measure unbroken, often folded, but many of thein too spread out, never curled, but always flattened, never brown, always deep green on their upper and gray-green on their under source, and uniform in that respect, seldom mottled in colour. They are thin and crisp, beautifully reticulated, and traversed longitudinally by a single fine vein on each side of the strong midrib. In mass they have a strong odour resembling that of tea, and when chewed they have a peculiar well-marked herbaceous taste, not disagreeable, followed, after a continuous chewing for some minutes by a gentle, pleasant sense of warmth in the mouth. Inferior specimens, besides differing in appearance from these, have a fainter odour, and do not occasion warmth in the mouth when chewed.

"Cuca has been subjected to chemical analysis, and found to contain a crystalline principle, to which naturally has been given the name of cocaine. But it is not my intention to enter here into the chemistry of the subject.

"Nor is the Botanical Society the fit place for discussing fully the experimental investigations which have been made into the physiological actions of cocaine, or of coca itself, further than as they bear on what has been said above upon that point, or on what is to follow as the account of my own observations. In that respect, the most important inquiry is that of Dr. Mantegazza of Milan, published in a prize essay, which has been noticed in the Őesterreichischce Zeitschrift fűr Praktische Heilkunde for November 1859.

"He found, by personal trials, that in small doses it promotes digestion, increases the frequency of the pulse, raises the animal heat, and accelerates respiration; that in a dose somewhat larger, there is added a facility of motion and desire for it, succeeded by a soothing effect; and that in a large dose, such as three drachms or upwards, it doubles the rate of the pulse, causes flashes of light, headache, strong tendency to muscular action, and great vigour of mind, succeeded by a state of pleasing, imaginative calm, described by him in brilliant colours, which resemble the poetical ravings of De Quincey, in representing the visionary musings of the opium-eater.

"A specimen of the plant is now in flower in the Edinburgh Botanic Garden (April 18th). It is well represented in an uncoloured engraving in Hooker's Companion to the Botanical Magazine, ii, 25, 1836.

"Were these effects the general rule, there would be more justice in the unfavourable representations of Pöppig than has been hitherto admitted. It must be allowed as some confirmation of Mantegazza's statement, that Weddell thought he occasionally observed hallucinations in the Coqueros of Peru, when under the influence of their dose; and that Von Tschudi saw effects which disposed him to compare Cuca with stramonium, an unequivocal narcotic poison. I scarcely think the recently ascertained deadly effects of the principle cocaine upon animals can be fairly added to the evidence in the same direction. It is true that experimental inquiries, and, among these, the most recent by Dr. Alexander Bennett, published in his thesis, and also as part of an experimental research carried on by a committee of the British Medical Association, prove that in small animals cocaine produces in an adequate dose paralysis of sensation, tetanic convulsions, and death. But he found the same effects to be caused by theine, caffeine, theobromine, and guaranine, the nearly identical crystalline principles of tea, coffee, chocolate, and the Brazilian guaranå; yet no one will imagine on that account, that the habitual use of these restoratives has any injurious influence on the health.

"At all events, however, the following experiments, with doses little short of those which are stated to have acted so extraordinarily in the case of Dr, Mantegazza, show results materially different from his, and prove that the leaves may be easily used by most, if not all, persons, so as to produce no unpleasant, unsafe, or even suspicious effects whatsoever. It must be acknowledged, nevertheless, from consideration of the whole facts recorded by good observers, and the opinions formed by competent judges, that, if Cuca is to be added to the restoratives of Europe—which seems not unlikely —it ought to be used at first with caution, and under close observation of its relative effect in several varieties of condition, such as age, sex, and constitution, rest and exercise, bodily and mental, dose and form, etc.

"My first trials were made in 1870, when I was not aware that anyone else in Europe had experimented with it. My specimen was sent to me by a London mercantile gentleman, Mr. Batchelor, six years before, and must therefore have been kept for seven years at least. The leaves had been excellently dried, flat, unbroken, and green; and they had been equally well preserved by sprinkling a little quick-lime among them before being shipped. Even in 1870 they were green, brittle, and strongly-scented. Two of my students, out of the habit of material exercise for five months, tired themselves thoroughly with a walk of sixteen miles in the month of April. They returned home at their dinner hour, having taken no food since a nine o'clock breakfast. They were very hungry, but refrained from food, and took each an infusion of two drachms of Cuca, made with the addition of five grains of carbonate of soda, which was added to imitate the Peruvian method of chewing the leaves along with a very small quantity of lime or plant ashes. I am satisfied, however, that any such addition is superfluous.

"Presently hunger left them entirely, all sense of fatigue soon vanished, and they proceeded to promenade Prince's Street for an hour; which they did with ease and pleasure. On returning home their hunger revived with great intensity; they made an excellent dinner ; they felt alert all the subsequent evening, slept soundly all night, and next morning awoke quite refreshed and active. One of them, in setting out for the evening promenade, felt very slightly giddy, as if he had taken just a little too much wine. But the other experienced no other sensation than the removal of fatigue, and ability for active exertion.

"Having subsequently received from Dr. Alexander Bennett a larger supply, obtained by him in Paris, I made farther trials in the spring of last year, 1875. This sample was more broken, less green, less scented than the other, less strong in taste, and scarcely producing any sense of warmth in the mouth when chewed. Obviously it was of lower quality. Ten of our students made trial of it under conditions precisely similar to those observed in the prior experiment; and they reported the results to me severally in writing. Their walks varied between twenty and thirty miles, and three cleared the latter distance on a rather hilly road at nearly mile pace over all. Two were unable to remark any distinct effect from the Cuca. Several felt decided, but only moderate relief from fatigue. Four experienced complete relief, like their predecessors in 1870; and one of these had walked thirty miles without any food. All found their hunger cease for a time; but shortly afterwards neither appetite nor digestion was at all impaired. No disagreeable effect was produced at the time or subsequently, except that a few felt a brief nausea after their dose, owing probably to the form of infusion in which it was taken.

"I then determined to make some careful personal trials with the scanty remains of my best specimen. For this purpose I thought it best to adopt the Peruvian method of chewing, but I discarded their lime and ashes. For not only was I unable to discover, in the nature, composition, or effects of the leaf, any chemical or physiological reason for such addition; but likewise I found that the Llipta, as the addition is called, which was presented to me with one of my specimens from Peru, has no alkaline or calcareous taste, and therefore cannot effect decomposition of the leaf while it is masticated. The result confirms the view I had thus taken.

"I had first to ascertain what amount of exercise was required to cause very thorough and permanent fatigue. At the same time, I made such observations on certain of the functions as seemed desirable and easily practicable. In the beginning of May, under a day temperature of 58 degrees , I walked fifteen miles in four stages, with intervals of half-an hour, at four-mile pace, without food or drink, after breakfast at half-past eight, and ending with a stage of six miles at half-past five in the afternoon. I had great difficulty in maintaining my pace through weariness towards the close, and was as effectually tired out as I remember ever to have been in my life, even after thirty miles at a stretch forty or fifty years before. Perspiration was profuse during every stage, particularly the last of all. I took the urine-solids every two hours, and found a decided increase of the hourly solids during the forenoon's exercise, and a decrease during the evening's rest after dinner. The pulse, naturally 62 at rest, was 110 on my arrival at home; and two hours later it was still 90. I was unfit for mental work in the evening, but slept soundly all night, and awoke next morning somewhat wearied and disinclined for active exercise, although otherwise quite well. Two days afterwards, I repeated this experiment, and obtained precisely the same results, except that the urine-solids were not so abundant during exercise as before, although my food had been precisely the same.

"Four days later, with precisely the same dietary, I walked sixteen miles in three stages of four, six, and six miles, with one interval of half-an-hour, and a second of an hour and a-half. During the last forty-five minutes of the second rest I chewed thoroughly eighty grains of my best specimen of Cuca, reserving forty grains more for use during the last stage. To make assurance double sure, I swallowed the exhausted fibre, which was my only difficulty. On completing the previous ten miles, I was fagged enough to look forward to the remaining six miles with considerable reluctance. I did not observe any sensible effect from the Cuca till I got out of doors, and put on my usual pace; when at once I was surprised to find that all sense of weariness had entirely fled, and that I could proceed not only with ease, but even with elasticity. I got over the six miles in an hour and a-half without difficulty, found it easy when done to get up a four-and-a-half mile pace, and to ascend quickly two steps at a time to my dressing-room, two floors upstairs; in short, had no sense of fatigue or other uneasiness whatsoever. During the last stage, I perspired as profusely as during the two previous walks.

"On arrival at home, the pulse was 90, and in two hours had fallen to 72 ; the excitement of the circulation being thus much less, and its subsidence more rapid, than after the same amount of exercise without Cuca. The urine-solids hourly were much the same while the exercise lasted as during exercise on the day of fifteen miles' walking without Cuca, although the breakfast dietary was precisely the same. During the evenings rest, the urine-solids were almost the same as during the preceding period of exercise—a fact which is capable of more interpretations than one.

"On arriving at home before dinner, I felt neither hunger nor thirst after complete abstinence from food and drink of every kind for nine hours; but on dinner appearing in half an hour, ample justice was done to it. Throughout the evening I was alert, and free from all drowsiness. Two hours of restlessness on going to bed I ascribed to the dose of two drachms being rather large; and after that I slept soundly, and awoke in the morning quite refreshed, and free from all sense of fatigue, and from all other uneasiness. Another effect, not unworthy of notice, was that a tenderness of the eyes, which for some years has rendered continuous reading a somewhat painful effort, was very much mitigated during all the evening.

"I reserved what remained of my good specimen of Cuca for further trial during my autumn holidays in the country. On September 15th, while residing at St. Fillans on Loch Earn, I ascended Ben Vorlich. The mountain is 3, 224 feet above the sea, and 2,900 feet above the highway on the loch-side. The ascent is for the most part easy, over first a rugged footpath, and then through short heather and short deep grass; but the final dome of 700 feet is very steep, and half of it among blocks and slabs of mica-slate, the abode of a few ptarmigan, of which a small covey was sprung in crossing the stony part. On the whole, no Highland mountain of the same height is more easily ascended. The temperature at the side of the lake was 62 degrees ; on the summit, 52 degrees. In consequence of misdirection, I had to descend an intervening slope on the way, so that the whole ascent was 3,000 feet perpendicular. I took two hours and a half to reach the summit, anl was so fatigued near the close, that it required considerable determination to persevere during the last 300 feet. I was richly rewarded, however, by an extremely clear atmosphere, and a magnificent mountainous panorama, of which the grandest object was Ben-Nevis, forty miles off, shown quite apart from other mountains, and presenting the whole of its great precipice edgeways to the eye. My companions, who, as well as I, were provided with an excellent luncheon, soon disposed of it satisfactorily; but I contented myself with chewing two-thirds of one drachm of Cuca leaves.

"We spent three-quarters of an hour at the top, during which I looked forward to the descent with no little distrust. On rising to commence it, however, although I had not previously experienced any sensible change, I at once felt that all fatigue was gone, and I went down the long descent with an ease like that which I used to enjoy in my mountainous rambles in my youth. At the bottom, I was neither weary, nor hungry, nor thirsty, and felt as if I could easily walk home four miles; but that was unnecessary. On arriving home at five o'clock, I still felt no fatigue, hunger, or thirst. At six, however, I made a very good dinner. During the subsequent evening, I was disposed to be busy, and not drowsy; and sound sleep during the night left me in the morning refreshed and ready for another day's exercise. I had taken neither food nor drink of any kind after breakfasting at half-past eight in the morning; but I continued to chew my Cuca till I finished the sixty grains when halfway down the mountain. I had not with me in the country any apparatus for observations on the renal secretion.

"Eight days afterwards, I repeated the experiment, but used ninety grains of Cuca. Being better acquainted with the way, no ground was lost by any intervening descent, so that the perpendicular height to be reached from the highway was 2,900 feet. I took two hours and a quarter to ascend, and on reaching the summit was extremely fatigued. The weather had changed, so that the temperature, 51 degrees at the loch-side, was 41 degrees at the top. A moderate breeze consequently caused so much chilliness that my party were glad to re-descend in half an hour, by which time I had consumed two-thirds of the Cuca, taking, as formerly, neither food nor drink. The effects were precisely the same, perhaps even more complete, for I easily made the descent without a halt in an hour and a quarter, covering at least four miles of rugged ground; and I walked homewards two miles of a smooth level road to meet my carriage. I then felt tired, because nearly three hours had elapsed since I consumed the Cuca, and in that time the Peruvians find it necessary to renew their restorative. But there was no more Cuca left, and I was tempted to substitute a draught of excellent porter. I suppose this indulgence led on to the unusual allowance of four glasses of wine during dinner, instead of one or none; and the two errors together, with possibly some discordance between Cuca and alcohol, were the probable cause of a restless feverish slumber during the early part of the night; but quiet sleep succeeded and I awoke quite refreshed and active next morning.

"One of my sons, who accompanied me on both occasions, used Cuca the first time, but also took luncheon on the summit. Though not in good condition for such work, he made it out without fatigue; and on the second occasion, when there was no more Cuca to give him, he felt decidedly the want of it when he reached the highway at the foot of the mountain.

"These trials have been described particularly, because I feel that,, without details, the general results, which may be now summarized, would scarcely carry conviction with them. These are the following. The chewing of Cuca removes extreme fatigue, and prevents it. Hunger and thirst are suspended; but eventually appetite and digestion are unaffected. No injury whatever is sustained at the time, or subsequently in occasional trials; but I can say nothing of what may or may not happen if it be used habitually. From sixty to ninety grains are sufficient for one trial; but some persons either require more, or are constitutionally proof against its restorative action. It has no effect on the mental faculties, so far as my own trials and other observations go, except liberating them from the dullness and drowsiness. which follow great bodily fatigue. I do not yet know its effect on mental fatigue purely. As to the several functions, it reduces the effect of severe protracted exercise in accelerating the pulse. It increases the saliva, which, however, may be no more than the effect of mastication. It does not diminish the perspiration, so far as I can judge. It probably lessens the hourly secretion of urine-solids. On this point I cannot yet speak with any confidence, because it appears to me that the investigation of the action of Paratriptics, or those substances which seem to lessen the wear and tear of the textures of the body in the exercise of their several functions, involves considerations and precautions which have escaped the attention of experimentalists on this interesting question, and which my own experiments hitherto have not taken completely into account.

"I have made no trials of the influence of Cuca on disease, or the consequences of disease. Some notices in the journals on this subject show that it is attracting attention ; but, so far as I see, it is a difficult one, and may prove extensive, and therefore it ought to fall into the hands of some able inquirer, who will be in no hurry to rush into print. I have been asked by correspondents in the south of England if Cuca will do good to a weak heart, to an old paralysis, to the feebleness of advancing age, etc. My reply has been, that I know nothing of all this, and that no one should use it medicinally, but under the advice and observation of his medical attendant.

"A more convenient form for use than that of a quid is very desirable. M. Laumaillé, who rode, or on very bad roads led, his bicycle 760 miles from Paris to Vienna in little more than twelve days, in the month of October, carried with him, as part of his scanty baggage, a small supply of the liqueur de coca, an Indian tonic, by which he was always able to assuage the sudden and painful hunger which sometimes accompanies continued exertion"

"Unfortunately, he gives us too little of his experience with it ; but he observes that, when about sixty miles from Vienna, " continuing his way along a road of fluid mire, fatigue and sleep at length told upon him, but the marvelous liqueur de coca again supported him and gave him strength". I have made by rule of thumb a very palatable liqueur, with only a fourth of rectified spirit, and containing in half-an-ounce the soluble part of sixty grains of leaves, but I have not yet tested its virtue. Pharmaceutical chemists, however, will soon solve this problem, and, it may be hoped, without looking for a patent.

# Appendix Two: Traditional Coca Leaf Medicines

## *Table of Traditional Coca Leaf Treatments & Cures*

Here's a little table I've put together to try to summarize some of known, traditionally respected natural medicine properties of Coca Leaf. I hope suggests that even if traditional medical wisdom and experience with Coca Leaf is only partially correct, a simple daily cup or two of fresh Coca leaf tea might help in some of these terrible diseases and conditions. Doesn't it make sense that fresh Coca Leaf for simple brewing as a medicinal tea, and quality natural medicines made from Coca Leaf, should be readily available without prescription to anyone who is suffering and in need?

| *Established Efficacy & Safety Of Coca Leaf (Not Cocaine) For Treatment and/or Cure in medical society journals and other publications and books by physicians from @ 1700-1900* | *Potential Efficacy & Safety of Coca Leaf for Treatment and/or Cure, based on pure guesswork, as of 2019 Some of these disorders are duplicated from the 1700-1900 list because they have emerged today as pandemics e.g. obesity and diabetes* |
|---|---|
| *(From Survey of 500+ American Physicians by Dr. Mortimer 1898-1900)* | *Stated/implied in Coca Leaf Medical/Scientific Literature 1700-1900* |
| *Drug Treatment (Opium/Alcohol)* | *Alzheimers/Dementia* |
| *Alcoholism* | *Obesity/Overweight* |
| *Anemia* | *ADHD* |
| *Angina Pectoris* | *Rheumatism* |
| *Asthma* | *Whole Body Inflammation* |
| *Brain Disorders* | *Diabetes* |
| *Bronchitis* | *Multiple Sclerosis* |
| *Convalescence/Wasting* | *Congestive Heart Failure* |
| *Debility/Overwork* | *Ischemic Heart Disease* |
| *Diabetes* | *Irritable Bowel Syndrome* |
| *Exhaustion/Fatigue* | *Crohn's* |
| *Fever* | *SIBO* |

| Heart Disorder | Neuromuscular Pain |
| --- | --- |
| Kidney Disorders | Peripheral Neuropathy |
| La Grippe (Flu) | Chronic Obstructive Pulmonary Disease |
| Lung Congestion | Pneumonia/Lower Respiratory Disease |
| Melancholia | Stroke |
| Muscle Pain | Hypertension |
| Nervous Exhaustion | |
| Neurasthesia | |
| Anorexia | |
| Obesity | |
| Sexual Exhaustion | |
| Shock | |
| Stomach & Intestinal Conditions | |
| Throat Conditions | |

I believe in the wisdom of the Indigenous Peoples of the Andes – "La Coca no es La Cocaine".

This of course is not a clever slogan, but the truth. However since those of us who live in the North have been deprived of any knowledge of medicinal Coca for over a century, we have no way of finding this truth for ourselves. Not so in Peru, Bolivia and now Uruguay. Check out this very interesting YouTube video on a company called IngaCoca. *https://tinyurl.com/yxvqlxym*

As you can see they are a Bolivian manufacturer of medicinal tonics and salves that combine the healing power of Coca Leaf extract with the healing power of a wide range of traditional medicinal herbs, many of them not familiar to us in the North. I hope that you find it worthwhile to take a few pages and consider the implications, and the potential, of the existence of this perfectly normal natural medicine company selling Coca Leaf medicines and tonics in a perfectly natural way in ordinary commerce. But not in America. Not yet.

Several things stand out about the IngaCoca website and the products that this company produces. First, while the healing power of Coca takes the lead role in all of their preparations, none of the preparations are simply Coca extract. The Indigenous Peoples of the Andes are not mono-maniacs when it comes to the medicinal properties of Coca. They don't see Coca as a stand-alone cure-all – although in some cases this great plant comes as close as anything else in nature's pharmacy to being a true panacea. So the products of IngaCoca always incorporate other, complementary medicinal herbs to form what they consider a healing solution for specific diseases and ailments.

Second, it's quite clear that not a single one of IngaCoca's products can possibly get you high – which is the excuse given by the USA and other authoritarian governments for banning trade in Coca Leaf. By the way, IMO there's nothing wrong with getting high, but Coca Leaf Tonic isn't going to do it for you. Unless, of course …..that happens to be the point.

The products that IngaCoca produces are proof positive that there is a vast range of medicinal applications of Coca Leaf that have nothing to do with recreational drug use. This is unlike Cannabis, which opponents of Medical Marijuana frantically point out – "Well, OK – it might possibly be good for you but MY GOD – IT GETS YOU HIGH!!!!" Venemous idiots, of course, but Cannabis does give them an opening while Coca Leaf does not.

As people have pointed out for hundreds of years, you could not chew enough Coca Leaves, or drink enough Coca tea, to get anything more than a mild coffee-style buzz. Coca Leaf is not about having fun – unless you think that preventing or curing dozens of nasty diseases and conditions is fun. Sounds pretty good to me.

The last thing that strikes me about the tonics and salves produced by IngaCoca is how many of the diseases and conditions that plague Americans and Europeans are NOT addressed by any of their products. None of their products are designed to address killer diseases like Congestive Heart Failure, Chronic Obstructive Pulmonary Disease, neurological diseases like MS and ALS, or Alzheimer's, that carry away tens of millions of Northern Hemisphere dwellers every year, and that there is plenty of evidence could be prevented treated, or even cured by having access to pure, natural Coca Leaf.

After pondering this for a few minutes it occurred to me – IngaCoca doesn't make Coca products to address these diseases because the people of the Andes don't need them. Take a took a look at the 50 leading causes of death in Peru and notice that the diseases that are true plagues upon the People of the North are minor factors in Peru and Bolivia. Sure there is some

Heart disease – almost all in urban dwellers. There is Diabetes – also mostly among urban dwellers. There is also a very low incidence of Lung disease. And – most interesting to me – there is zero Dementia/Alzheimer's. Nowhere in the 50 leading causes of death in the Andes.

Does that suggest something to you about our toxic environment, and most likely our industrialized food chain, in the North?

IngaCoca are pioneers, and deserve great credit for demonstrating that their national treasure is far, far more than the white powder that gives the governments of the world an excuse to make Coca Leaf illegal. We all understand that this is about protecting the global Pharmaceutical industry, and giving free reign to the Cartels and their Big Bank money launderers and co-conspirators, and to a few less obvious stakeholders like the anti-drug police bureaucracies.

Perhaps, in time and with increasing enlightenment of the people, a few legislators in the US or elsewhere will grow at least some tiny Cojones and do something about this farce which is actually a death sentence for millions of people whose interests they claim to care about. Without access to pure, natural medicines, and condemned to use only the toxic products of the greedheads who run Pig Pharma, that is exactly the result of the "War on Drugs" – mandatory death sentences for millions.

In the meanwhile I would like to encourage readers of this book who live in countries that are enlightened enough to recognize the difference between Coca Leaf medicines and Cocaine to look into helping IngaCoca reach people in your country with its products. This could be not only a humanitarian effort, but perhaps a nice little opportunity too.

### *IngaCoca Medicines & Commentary*

### *Coca Leaf For Asthma?*

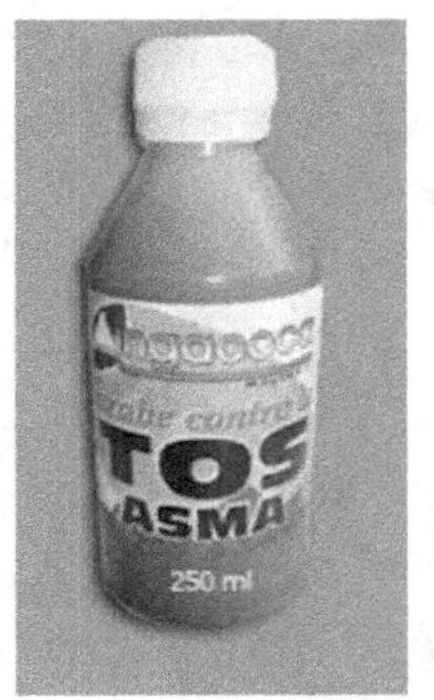


IngaCoca says:

"This Tonic Is Effective For: Cough, Asthma , Bronchitis , Tonsillitis
Composition: A natural compound of Coca, Wirawira , Cardosanto and Eucalyptus."
"Wirawira is known as a remedy for coughs, bronchitis, hoarseness, high fever, stomach ache, indigestion, sores and wounds, inflamed throat, colds and flu. This herb has proven antibiotic and antiviral activity."
"The flowers of Cardo Santo are a natural remedy for anemia, loss of appetite, migraines and inflammatory conditions."

*"Asthma is an exceedingly unfortunate affliction which may exhibit no local signs between the attacks. It is occasioned by a spasm of the minute tubes set up reflexly either by trouble in the upper air passages, or wholly from a nervous influence, and an attack is often precipitated by worry or some unusual nervous strain. The source of trouble is well prevented by the judicious use of Coca, not only acting beneficially upon the mucous membrane, but through a sedative influence upon nervous tissue and as a tonic support to the muscular system generally."* (in) W. Mortimer Golden, **History Of Coca,** 1901

## Coca Leaf Tonic For The Prostate?

IngaCoca Says:

"This Tonic Is Effective For: Prostate, Bladder inflammation."

Composition: Natural therapeutic compound of COCA from Kishuara , Yareta and Flower Of The Valley . It is used in pain, obstruction and hypertrophy of the prostate, and inflammation of the urethra and bladder.

Yareta or llareta is a flowering plant in the family Apiaceae native to South America. It resembles a mound of green moss rather than a flowering plant, and is found primarily in remote, arid regions of the Altiplano region of Bolivia.

## Coca Leaf Tonic For Nervous Exhaustion & Anxiety?

IngaCoca Says: "This Tonic Is Effective For: The Nerves
Composition: A natural composition of Coca, Matico, Totongil , Valerian and Rosemary possess excellent therapeutic properties which facilitates oxygenation to the brain."

"Use as an Antidepressant, for Stress, Nervous Tension, Insomnia, and Dizziness."

"Matico has strong styptic properties are due to the volatile oil, and it is used for arresting hemorrhages, as a local application to ulcers, in genito-urinary complaints, atonic diarrhoea, dysentery, etc. In Peru it is also considered an aphrodisiac. It is effective as a topical application to slight wounds, bites of leeches, or after the extraction of teeth. The under surface of the leaf is preferred to the powder for this purpose."

"Totongil, or Melissa, is also known as lemon balm, lemongrass or lemon leaf. Totongil is used as a tea as a natural tranquilizer with anti-spasmodic properties. It is used in the resuscitation of fainting and as a natural painkiller. Other medicinal properties include treatment of Tachycardia or palpitations of nervous origin, where lemon balm calms the heart muscle and restores normal rhythm to the heart."

*"In the way of medication and as an adjunct to the food I know of no better remedy than Coca, preferably the original wine of Coca prepared by Mariani. In this the properties of Coca are appropriately preserved by some special method of manufacture, while the mild wine adds a temporary stimulation which is enhanced by the more permanent influence of the Coca."* (in) W. Mortimer Golden, ***The History Of Coca***, 1901

## *Coca Leaf Tonic For Gut Disorders?*

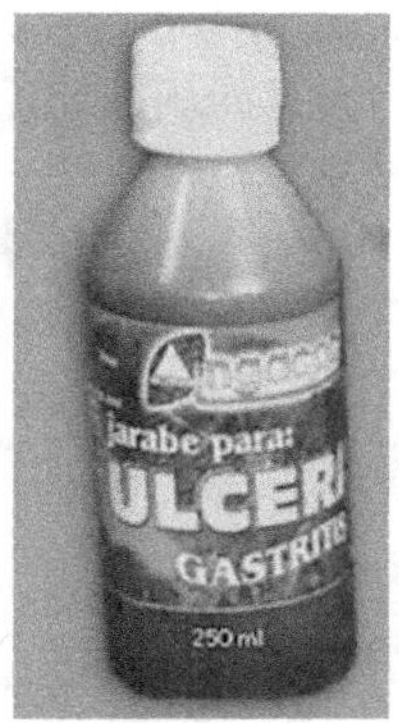


IngaCoca Says: "This Tonic Is Effective For: Ulcers" Composition: A natural composition of Coca, phasa, matico, mauve and thusca. Possesses therapeutic properties for stomach ulcers and gastritis; helps prevent ulcerative disorders that affect the gut.

*"From another point of view, M. Laffont adds, that the dynamogenic action of the active principles of Coca on the smooth-fibered muscles "indicates its use in the list of atonic gastro-intestinal diseases, flatulent dyspepsia, dilatation of the stomach, paresis of the intestines, of the bladder, etc."* History of Coca, 1901

## *Coca Leaf Tonic For Obesity?*

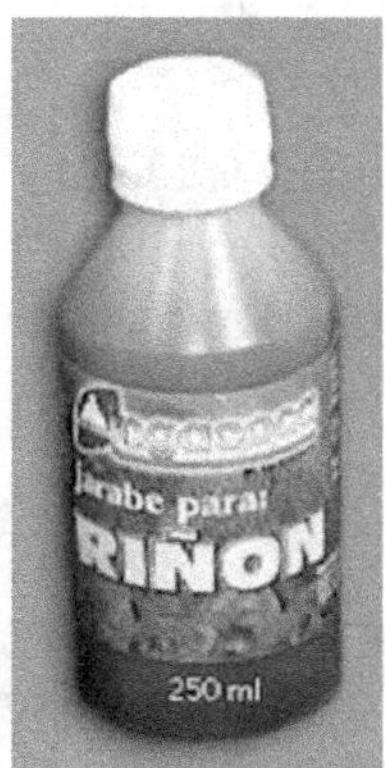


IngaCoca Says: "This Tonic Is Effective For: Weight Loss"

"Composition: natural composition Coca, chick (?), lupine and others.

Contains Egnonina. Therapeutic for metabolizing fats and carbohydrates, eliminating obesity, purifying the blood and regulating cholesterol."

*"After Moreno y Maïz, Dr. Gazeau, in 1870, studied the stimulating effect of Coca on nutrition, and found that it increased the pulse and respiration, assisted digestion, increased urinary excretion, and strengthened the nervous system. This author arrived at the conclusion that Coca prolongs life and promotes muscular energy. He advises its use, locally, for stomatitis, gingivitis, aphthous ulceration, and generally for painful and difficult digestion, gastric disturbance in phthisis, and also for obesity."* History of Coca, 1901

### *Coca Leaf Tonic For Diabetes?*

IngaCoca Says: "This Tonic Is Effective For: Anti-Diabetic"

Composition: Natural extract of Coca, sage, lupine and dandelion, forms a therapeutic substance that normalizes the functioning of the pancreas, regulating the secretion of natural insulin.

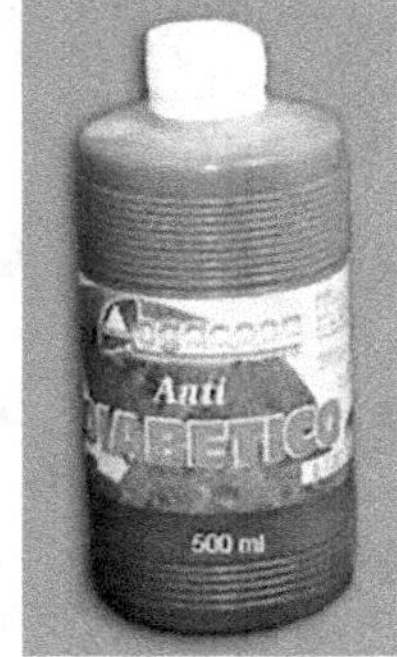

*"Coca in the conversion of these soluble products into less soluble glycogen and proteids, and indicates a possible application of Coca to the relief of diabetes and albuminuria, disorders in which it has already been employed empirically with advantage."* (in) **History of Coca** by W. Golden Mortimer, MD, 1901

### *Coca Leaf Tonic For Physical/Mental Energy?*

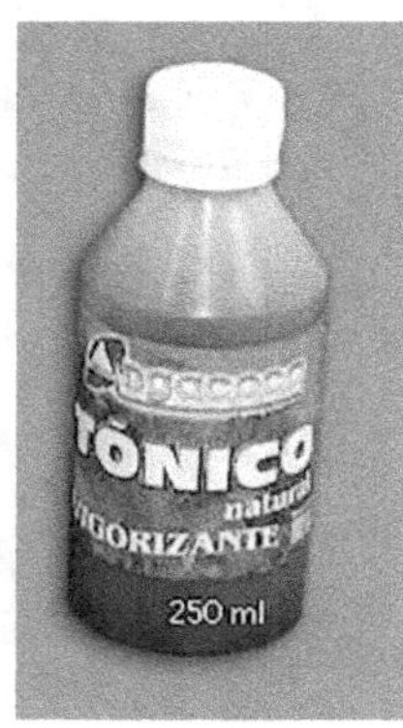

IngaCoca Says:

"This Tonic Is Effective For: Energy"

Composition : The natural essence of: Coca, Alfalfa, Beet Root , Spinach and Abeja honey.

Works effectively as a powerful stimulant of blood, and muscle system develops more force if energy is depleted, in cases of Hemorrhage, Anemia, diminished Mental Activity, Sexual Function, and/or Appetite."

*" Manuel Fuentes, of Lima, said: '"Whatever may be thought of the explanation, the fact is that the human body acquires by the continued use of Coca an athletic constitution, capable of resisting, among privations and misery, the severest fatigue as well as the inclemency of the weather. Experience and scientific analysis reveal to us in Coca the most tonic plant in the vegetable kingdom. This precious shrub unites in itself all the virtues which are separately met with in the large number of vegetables comprised under the general name of "tonic plants."*

### *Coca Leaf Tonic For Liver & Kidney Function?*

IngaCoca Says: "This Tonic Is Effective For: Liver & Kidneys"

Composition : Coca, Chanca Stone, Sarsaparilla, Artichoke, Horsetail And Ortiga.

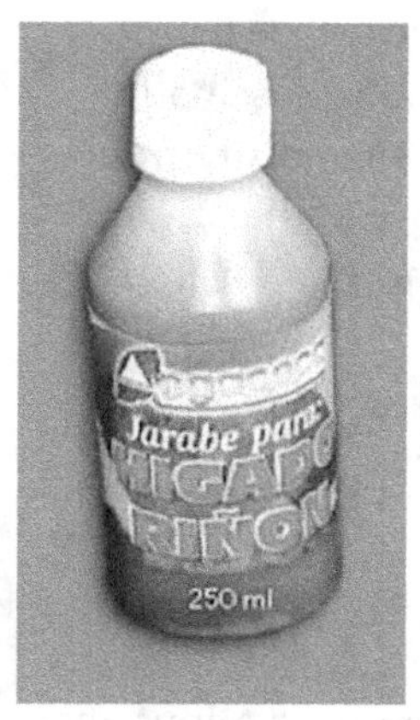

This tonic has therapeutic properties that reduce inflammation and clean the excess fat from the Liver and Kidney and also facilitate filtration. Ortiga (ortiga verde) is a member of the stinging nettle family of herbs. The Nettle family has a worldwide reputation as an effective treatment for purifying the blood, fighting inflammation and internal infections, and promoting digestive health.

*"If the hypothesis be true that Coca frees the blood of products of waste, this affords ample explanation of properties attributed to Coca which have hitherto appeared phenomenal, and its wide-spread usefulness and seemingly contradictory action over a host of apparently dissimilar conditions may be well understood. Whether the relief sought be for a simple vocal strain, for rheumatism, or for mountain sickness, nervous irritability or muscular fatigue, the conditions are of common origin. Coca simply makes better blood and a healthy blood makes healthy tissue."* (in) History of Coca, 1901

### In Summary

OK, maybe IngaCoca's Tonics work as claimed and maybe they don't – IngaCoca didn't exist that last time I was in the southern Andes a very long time ago. But every one of the conditions for which they have a tonic is a condition that is documented in the old books as being treatable or curable in some cases by the right tincture or tonic of Coca leaf and medicinal herbs.

I can't resist this last little quote from a doctor whose lifetime work was treating anemia in the mid-1800's:

*"In anemia, connected with chronic pulmonary affections without fever, and in anemia accompanied by gastralgic pains, Coca will have an excellent effect. The stimulating properties of Coca can also be admirably utilized in those intermediate states of impaired health which are not yet anemia, but must in the end become so — the cerebral weakness due to excess of work or pleasure, the exhaustion from which the inhabitants of large cities suffer, from irregularities of diet and imperfect hygiene due to their positions and surroundings."* (in) History of Coca, 1901

Sounds like we could all use a little Coca tea in our lives, doesn't it?

# Bibliography: Your Keys To Ancient Knowledge

This Coca Bibliography will link you to some of the most fascinating books on Coca that I've found in searching the vast Coca literature from past centuries. I have created a 'tinyurl' for each reference to the original text, which in most cases can be downloaded as a pdf for your leisurely exploration.

The quickest way to use the Tinyurl to access any of the references is to keep *https://tinyurl.com/* available on your computer or phone then when you see a reference you want to browse just paste *https://tinyurl.com/* into your browser, enter your selected 8 digit letter/number combination at the end, and you're there – deep in the past reading someone with interesting points of view and often challenging, always interesting observations about Coca and Mama Coca, the Andean cultures and environments, the traditions and practices of the people of those times and places where Coca flourished as a natural part of a good life even under often difficult conditions.

I hope that you enjoy following some of these links to the voices of people from the distant past and their sometimes brilliant, sometimes offensive, and always interesting things to say about the world of Mama Coca as they experienced it.

> *A note: some of these old books and documents are pretty rough. The racism and brutality of our own times have deep roots in history, and a lot of it is right here in these voices. To extract the value of their knowledge you have to set aside their occasional insanity and just love their weirdness.*

## 300 Years Of Coca: Experiences & Worldviews

ACOSTA, JOSE DE: Historia natural y moral de las Indias; Sevilla, 1588. Translated into French by Robert Regnault, Paris, 1616. Translated into English by Clements R. Markham, C.B., F.R.S. (Hakluyt Society), London.

*https://tinyurl.com/yytvzd8y*

ALLEN, TIMOTHY F., A. M., M.D.: Encyclopedia of Pure Materia Medica; III, pp. 369-381; 8vo.

*https://tinyurl.com/y58jc2z5*

ALMS, H.: Die Wirkung des Cocains auf die peripherischen Nerven; Archiv für Physiologic, [Suppl-band.] p. 293; Leipzig, 1886.

*https://tinyurl.com/y4dq8xzw*

ANREP, B. VON: Ueber die physiologische Wirkung des Cocaïn; Archiv für die gesammte Physiologic, XXI; Bonn, 1880. Also Journal Medecine de Chirurgie, et de Pharmacologie, IXX; Bruxelles, 1880.

*https://tinyurl.com/yygjq2ne*

ANSTIE, FRANCIS E.: Stimulants and Narcotics; Their Mutual Relations, with special researches on the Action of Alcohol, Ether and Chloroform on the Vital Organism; 8vo. ; Philadelphia, 1865.

*https://tinyurl.com/yyvuwjb9*

ARANGO, A. P.: Note sur la Coca; Bulletin general de therapeutique, IXXX; Paris, 1871. (Ed. Note – you will have to enter a 'Capture" number to enter the archives and access this document. The Capture number for this citation is #462)

*https://tinyurl.com/y5qa4q3r*

ARRIGA, JOSE DE: Estirpacion de la Idolatria del Peru; Lima, 1621.

*https://tinyurl.com/y2wp5ck5*

AUBREY, GEORGES: Contribution a l'etude de la Coca du Pérou, et de la cocaïne. 2 pi., 4to. ; Nancy, 1885.

*https://tinyurl.com/y6nhkdpt*

BAKER, A. R.: The Coca Leaf and Its Alkaloid; Cincinnati Lancet- Clinic (n. s.), XIII; Cincinnati, 1884.

*https://tinyurl.com/y3mqm8h3*

BALFOUR, JOHN HUTTON, M.D.: A Manual of Botany; London, 1849.

https://tinyurl.com/y3jeay3j

BARTHOLOW, ROBERTS, M.A., M.D., LL.D. : A Practical Treatise on Materia Medica and Therapeutics; 5 ed.; New York, 1885.

https://tinyurl.com/y3h6y27y

BEARD, GEORGE M., M.D.:: Treatise on Nervous Exhaustion; New York, 1880.

https://tinyurl.com/y3fkoo69

BEARD, GEORGE M., M.D.:: Sexual Neurasthenia; Edited by A. D. Rockwell, A.M., M.D., 2 ed.; New York, 1886.

https://tinyurl.com/y32vhf2v

BEAU, J. H. S.: Traité de la Dyspepsie; 8vo.; Paris, 1866.

https://tinyurl.com/yygawhbe

BELL, JOHN: Regimen and Longevity; Philadelphia, 1842.

https://tinyurl.com/y2mgmxfo

BENTLEY, W. H.: Erythroxylon Coca; Therapeutic Gazette; (n. s.), I; Detroit, 1880. (Ed. Note: Incomplete text of article)

https://tinyurl.com/y3mkh7q6

BENTLEY and TRIMEN: Medicinal Plants; 4 vols., 8vo.; London, 1880.

https://tinyurl.com/yx9xnvrb

BERNARD, CLAUDE: Nouvelle Fonction du Foie; Paris, 1853.

https://tinyurl.com/y6b4nobm

BERNARD, CLAUDE: Leçons sur le Diabète ; Paris, 1877.

https://tinyurl.com/y5hbhzlc

BERNARD, W. : Observations on the effects of Cuca leaves; British Medical Journal, I; London, 1876.

https://tinyurl.com/y2aprzjw

BEUGNIER-CORBEAU : Recherches historiques, expérimentales et thérapeutiques sur la Coca et son alcaloide; Bulletin general de thérapeutique, CVII; Paris, 1884.

https://tinyurl.com/y2usw6cn

BIBEA, DR. ERNST FREYHERR VON: Die Narkotischen Genussmittel und der Mensch. (Art. Coca), pp. 151-174; Nürnberg, 1855.

https://tinyurl.com/y3msy88v

BICHAT, M. F. X.: Physiological Researches on Life and Death. Translated by F. Gold, London, 1799.

https://tinyurl.com/yxp5td9k

BIGNON, A: Note on the Properties of Coca and Cocaine; [Nouveaux Remèdes] ; Pharmaceutical Journal and Transactions; Sept. 26, London, 1885.

https://tinyurl.com/y3g73x62

BOCQUILLON, H.: Manuel d'Histoire Naturelle Médicale; 12mo. ; Paris, 1871.

https://tinyurl.com/y4s8dgwx

BRAID, JAMES: Neurypnology, or the Rationale of Nervous Sleep considered in Relation with Animal Magnetism; London, 1843.

https://tinyurl.com/y2dpa9aw

BRINTON, DANIEL G., M.D., LL.D.: Myths of the New World; 12mo.; Philadelphia, 1868.

https://tinyurl.com/yxecthsy

BROADBENT, SIR W. H., M.D., F.R.C.P.: The Pulse; London.

https://tinyurl.com/y2y26rbk

BROWNE, LENNOX, and EMIL BEHNKE: Voice, Song and Speech 2 ed.; 1886.

https://tinyurl.com/y2psh7h5

BROWNE, PATRICK, M.D.: The Civil and Natural History of Jamaica; folio, p. 278; London, 1756.

https://tinyurl.com/y3b6a37t

BRUCE, J. MITCHELL, M.D.: Materia Medica, 12mo.; Philadelphia, 1884.

https://tinyurl.com/y2qd6q3p

BRUNTON, T. LAUDER, M.D., F.R.S., etc.: Pharmacology, Therapeutics and Materia Medica; Adapted to the U. S. Pharmacopeia by Francis H. Williams, M.D., 8vo.; Philadelphia, 1885.

https://tinyurl.com/y62zm2g3

CAUDWELL, EBER, M.D.: The physiological action of Cuca and cucaine; British Medical Journal, Jan. 3, London, 1885.

https://tinyurl.com/y36k3kqn

CHRISTISON, SIR ROBERT, M.D. : The effects of Cuca or Coca: The leaves of Erythroxylon Coca; Address before the Royal Botanical Society of Edinburgh, April 13, 1876, on the restoration and preservative virtues of the Coca leaf against bodily fatigue; Pharmaceutical Journal and Transactions, (3 s.), VI; also British Medical Journal, I; London, 1876.

https://tinyurl.com/y3cupmds

COCHET, ALEXANDRE: Note sur la culture et ses usages de la Coca; Journal de chimie médicale, de pharmacie, de toxicologie, VIII; p. 475; Paris, 1832.

https://tinyurl.com/y4296934

COLE, R. FITZ-ROY: The Peruvians at Home; 12mo. \; London, 1884.

https://tinyurl.com/yy2y5alt

COLMAN, CHARLES: Myths of the Hindus. 1832

https://tinyurl.com/y2vsbrs6

COLOMBE, GABRIEL: Etude sur la Coca et les sels de cocaine; 4to.; Paris, 1885.

https://tinyurl.com/y47b2ll3

CORNING, J. LEONARD, M.D.: Brain Exhaustion; 8vo.; New York, 1884.

https://tinyurl.com/yxdbkt8k

CORNING, J. LEONARD, M.D: Brain-Rest: A disquisition on the curative properties of prolonged sleep; 2 ed., 12mo.; New York, 1885.

https://tinyurl.com/y4btcv68

CORNING, J. LEONARD, M.D: Local Anaesthesia in General Medicine and Surgery; 8vo.; New York, 1886.

https://tinyurl.com/y34bkc6d

COWLEY, ABRAHAM, M.D.: Poems; Four Books of Plants; London, 1721.

https://tinyurl.com/yysz9ds4

CURTIS, CARLTON C. A.M., Ph.D.: A Text-Book of General Botany; 8vo.; London, 1897.

https://tinyurl.com/y3clnjtq

DARWIN, CHARLES: Narrative of the Surveying voyages of His Majesty's ships Adventure and Beagle between the years 1826-1836; 3 vols., 8vo.; London, 1839.

https://tinyurl.com/y2olgu7y

DARWIN, CHARLES: On the Origin of Species by means of Natural Selection; 6 ed., 8vo.; London, 1872.

https://tinyurl.com/y27d35mh

DARWIN, CHARLES: The Expression of the Emotions in Man and Animals; 8vo.; London, 1872.

https://tinyurl.com/yxhxp9pp

DARWIN, CHARLES: Insectivorous Plants; 8vo.; London, 1875.

https://tinyurl.com/y58am5zy

DARWIN, CHARLES: The Movements and Habits of Climbing Plants; 2 ed.; London, 1875.

https://tinyurl.com/yxm7oet5

DARWIN, CHARLES: The different forms of flowers on plants of the same Species; 8vo. ; London, 1877.

https://tinyurl.com/yy6jmtuq

DARWIN, CHARLES: The Descent of Man; 2 vols., 2 ed., 8vo.; London, 1883.

https://tinyurl.com/yxqkom54

DARWIN, CHARLES: The Variation of Animals and Plants under domestication; 2 vols., 2 ed., 8vo.; London, 1885.

https://tinyurl.com/y5ky2xw9

DAY, ALFRED: Treatise on Harmony; 1845.

https://tinyurl.com/yy9lg778

DEANE, JOHN B : Serpent Worship. 1833

https://tinyurl.com/y6d4vc2y

DE CANDOLLE, ALPHONSE: Origin of Cultivated Plants; 12mo. ; New York, 1886.

https://tinyurl.com/y5h58j78

DE CANDOLLE, PYRAMUS: Prodromus systematis naturalis, regni vegetabilis; I, pp. 574-575, 8vo. ; Paris, 1824.

https://tinyurl.com/yyqlow6n

DELANO, AMASA: Narrative of Voyages and Travels in the Northern and Southern Hemispheres: Comprising Three Voyages around the World; 8vo.; Boston, 1817.

https://tinyurl.com/y6y98ebk

DEMARLE, L. G.: Sur la Coca; 4to; Paris, 1862.

https://tinyurl.com/yxnm9mpx

D'ISRAELI, ISAAC: Curiosities of Literature; (Art. Tea, Coffee and Chocolate), London, 1823.

https://tinyurl.com/y4o5cf63

D'ORBIGNY, ALCIDE DESSALINES : L'Homme Américain, 2 vols. Same: Voyage dans Amérique méridionale; Relation historique, II; 9 vols., 4to.; Paris, 1839-45.

https://tinyurl.com/y3wdcrb3

DUJARDIN-BEAUMETZ : Diseases of the Stomach and Intestines; Translated by E. P. Kurd, M.D.; Svo.; New York, 1886.

https://tinyurl.com/yxdtbbv6

DUJARDIN-BEAUMETZ: New Medications; (Art. Coca), Translated by E. P. Hurd, M.D.; Detroit, 1886.

https://tinyurl.com/y3b7t2c5

DYER, THOMAS F.T.: The Folk-Lore of Plants.

https://tinyurl.com/y2yd25nn

EDSON, CYRUS, M.D.: La Grippe and its Treatment; 12mo.; New York, 1891.

https://tinyurl.com/y26q7zwa

EMMET, THOMAS ADDIS, M.D. : The Principles and Practice of Gynaecology; (Art. Principles of General Treatment), Philadelphia, 1879.

https://tinyurl.com/y497ekon

FERGUSON, JAMES: Rude Stone Monuments.

https://tinyurl.com/y6cblact

FITZ GERALD, EDWARD A.: The Highest Andes; 8vo.; New York, 1899.

https://tinyurl.com/y6o7b83a

FRANKLAUSER, W.: Coca as a stimulant; American Medical and Surgical Bulletin, VII; New York, 1894.

https://tinyurl.com/yyhs2lgg

FREUD, S: Beiträge zur Kenntniss der Cocawirkung; Wiener medizinische Wochenschrift, XXXV; Vienna, 1885.

https://tinyurl.com/y2mvdxej

FREUD, S: Ueber Coca; Neu durchgeseh. u. verm. Sep.-Abdr. aus dem Centralblatt für die gesammte Therapie; Vienna, 1885

https://tinyurl.com/y677pklf

FREUD, S: Bemerkungen über Cocaïnsucht und Cocaïnfurcht; Wiener Medizinische Wochenschrift, XXXVII; 929-932; Vienna, 1887.

https://tinyurl.com/y26lrxsh

GARCILASSO DE LA VEGA: The First Part of the Royal Commentaries of the Yncas; 1609. Translated and edited with notes and Introduction by Clements R. Markham, C.B., F.R.S. (Hakluyt Society); 8vo.; London, 1871.

https://tinyurl.com/yxqbyvs4

GILLESPIE, A. LOCKHART: The Natural History of Digestion; 12mo.; London, 1898.

https://tinyurl.com/y6ssadzu

GRIFFITHS, A. B., Ph.D., F.R.C.S., etc.: Researches on Micro-Organisms; 12mo.; London, 1891.

https://tinyurl.com/y65vplsh

GUBLER, ADOLPHE, M.D.: Principles and Methods of Therapeutics. English translation; Philadelphia, 1881.

https://tinyurl.com/yxoz8kbk

GUIBOURT, JEAN BAPTISTE: Histoire naturelle des drogues simples, III, p. 545, 4me edit., 8vo.; Paris, 1850.

https://tinyurl.com/y4kroncn

HAIG, ALEXANDER, M.A., M.D., etc.: Uric Acid as a Factor in the Causation of Disease; 4 ed., 8vo. ; London, 1897.

https://tinyurl.com/y4pozac8

HALL, CAPTAIN BASIL (Royal Navy) : Extracts from a Journal written on the coasts of Chili, Peru and Mexico in the years 1820- 21-22; 2 vols.; London, 1825.

https://tinyurl.com/y5veajmx

HAMMOND, WILLIAM A., M.D.: Sleep and its Derangements; Philadelphia, 1869.

https://tinyurl.com/y5kh7ptu

HAMMOND, WILLIAM A., M.D: Diseases of the Nervous System; 8vo.; New York, 1886.

https://tinyurl.com/yxwl24ax

HAWEIS, REV. HUGH R.: Music and Morals; 12mo.; London, 1873.

https://tinyurl.com/yxedqw3d

HEINIGKE, DR. CARL: Pathogenetic Outlines of Homœopathic Drugs; New York, 1880.

https://tinyurl.com/y34ut86l

HELMHOLTZ, HERMANN, L.F.: On the sensations of tone as a physiological basis of the theory of music. Translated by Alexander J. Ellis; 3 ed.; London, 1895.

https://tinyurl.com/y4ha8fwf

HELPS, ARTHUR: The Spanish Conquest in America and Its Relations to the History of Slavery and to the Government of Colonies; 4 vols.; London, 1855.

https://tinyurl.com/y33mpf9o

HEMPEL, CHARLES J., M.D.: Materia Medica and Therapeutics; 8vo.; Chicago, 1880.

https://tinyurl.com/y5l7mx77

HERNDON, WILLIAM LEWIS, and LARUNER GIBBON, Lieutenants, U.S.N. Exploration of the Valley of the Amazon; made under Direction of the Navy Department; 2 vols., 8vo.; Washington, 1853

https://tinyurl.com/y4jd7cjr

HUMBOLDT, ALEXANDRE DE, et AIME BONPLAND: Personal Narrative of Travels to the Equinoctial Regions of the New Continent, etc., during the Years 1799-1804; 8 vols.; London, 1849.

https://tinyurl.com/y4gvp5z2

INWARDS, RICHARD: The Temple of the Andes; London, 1884.

https://tinyurl.com/y3m6oj5m

JACKSON, JOHN R., A.L.S.: Commercial Botany of the Nineteenth Century; 12mo.; London, 1890.

https://tinyurl.com/y26483kq

KAVANAGH, MORGAN P.: Origin of Language and Myths. 1871

https://tinyurl.com/y49fh7a7

KELLER, FRANZ: The Amazon and Madeira Rivers; 4to. ; New York, 1874.

https://tinyurl.com/y6mwqy95

KING, C. W.: The Gnostics and their Remains, Ancient and Medieval; London, 1864.

https://tinyurl.com/y63ldd49

KIRKES: Handbook of Physiology: by W. Morrant Baker, F.R.C.S., and Vincent Dormer Harris, M.D.; 11 ed.; London, 1884.

https://tinyurl.com/y5pr6doy

KRAFT-EBING, R. VON: Psychopathia Sexualis; Translated by Charles Gilbert Chaddock, M.D.; 8vo.; Philadelphia, 1892.

https://tinyurl.com/y22ujagm

LABORDE, J. V.: Note préliminaire sur l'action physiologique de la cocaïne et ses sels; Tribune medicale. XVI; Paris, 1884.

https://tinyurl.com/y6tpyhda

LE PLONGEON, AUGUSTUS: Sacred Mysteries among the Mayas and Quiches, 11,500 years ago; 8vo.; New York, 1886.

https://tinyurl.com/yyv3e857

LIEBIG, JUSTUS: Animal Chemistry or Chemistry in its Application to Physiology and Pathology; London, 1843.

https://tinyurl.com/y4r7a9yb

LINDLEY, JOHN, Ph.D.: The Vegetable Kingdom; 8vo.; London, 1853.

https://tinyurl.com/yxpll2n9

LUDEWIG, ERNST: Literature of American Aboriginal Languages. 1858

https://tinyurl.com/yxqfra8f

MAISCH, JOHN M: A Manual of Organic Materia Medica, 5 ed., 12mo., Philadelphia, 1892.

https://tinyurl.com/yxm9thxo

MARKHAM, CLEMENTS. C. B., F. R. S.: Cuzco; a Journey to the Ancient Capital of Peru; With an Account of the History, Language, Literature and Antiquities of the Incas, with Illustrations and Map, 8vo.; London, 1856. (Mr. Markham translated and edited most of the works of the earlier Peruvian historians which are published by the Hakluyt Society, London.)

https://tinyurl.com/yxfcpzyu

MARKHAM, CLEMENTS. C. B., F. R. S: Travels in Peru and India, with Maps and Illustrations, 8vo.; London, 1862.

https://tinyurl.com/y3yyqzum

MARKHAM, CLEMENTS. C. B., F. R. S: A Memoir of the Lady Ana de Osorio, Countess of Chinchon and Vice-Queen of Peru, with a plea for the correct spelling of the Chinchona genus; Map and Illustrations, 4to. ; London, 1874.

https://tinyurl.com/y239pyxt

MARKHAM, CLEMENTS. C. B., F. R. S: A History of Peru; Chicago, 1892.

https://tinyurl.com/yyojc5jl

MAYO, ROBERT: Mythology of Pagan World. 1815

https://tinyurl.com/y3onhtne

MITCHELL, S. WEIR, M.D.: Fat and Blood, 4 ed., 12mo.; Philadelphia, 1884.

https://tinyurl.com/y4v39qsw

MOLINA, CHRLSTOVAL DE: The Fables and Rites of the Yncas (MSS. 1570-1584). Translated and edited by Clements R. Markham, C.B., F.R.S. (Hakluyt Society); London, 1873. (The original Peruvian manuscript was translated and published in French by Ternaux Compans in 1840.)

https://tinyurl.com/y428u3ac

MUELLER, BARON FEKU.: Select Extra Tropical Plants readily eligible for Industrial Culture or Naturalization; 7 ed., 8vo.; Melbourne, 1888.

https://tinyurl.com/y5q3njk5

MURCHISON, CHARLES: Clinical lectures on Diseases of the Liver, 3 ed.; New York, 1885.

https://tinyurl.com/y2p8bhv7

NADAILLAC, MARQUIS DE: Prehistoric America. Translated by N. D'Anvers, edited by W. H. Doll, 8vo.; London, 1885.

https://tinyurl.com/y66vrndr

NADAILLAC, MARQUIS DE: Manners and Monuments of Prehistoric Peoples. Translated by N. D'Anvers, 8vo.; New York, 1892.

https://tinyurl.com/y5ofpnva

NEUDORFER J.: Die Coca; Allgemeiner Milärzte Zeitung; 377-380; Vienna, 1870.

https://tinyurl.com/y6359dgh

NOVY, FREDERICK G., M.S.: Cocaine and Its Derivatives; 12 mo.; Detroit, 1887.

https://tinyurl.com/y6d7tsqo

OTT, ISAAC: Physiological action of the leaves of the Erythroxylon Coca on the excretion of urine; Medical Times, I; Philadelphia, 1870-71.

https://tinyurl.com/y3zf88rm

PALMER, E. R. : Coca in fatigue; American Practitioner, XXXI; 69- 74, Louisville, 1885.

https://tinyurl.com/y5juktuw

PAVY, F. W., M.D., F.R.S.: A Treatise on Food and Dietetics, 2 ed., 8vo.; London, 1875.

https://tinyurl.com/y6zdz8jj

PRESCOTT, WILLIAM H. : History of the Conquest of Peru, with a Preliminary View of the Civilization of the Incas; Edited with notes by John Foster Kirk, 2 vols.; Philadelphia, 1848.

https://tinyurl.com/y4ph6c8t

RAIMONDI, DON ANTONIO: El Perú; 8vo., 3 vols.; Lima, 1874. (An elaborate work of Peruvian history and customs. Since the death of the author the Geographical Society has undertaken its completion.)

https://tinyurl.com/y62houly

ROBINSON, BEVERLEY, M.D.: Heart Strain and Weak Heart; Medical Record, Feb. 26, New York, 1887.

https://tinyurl.com/yxjo8kcz

RUSBY, HENRY H., M.D: Coca at home and abroad; Therapeutic Gazette; (3 s.), IV; pp. 158-165; also 303-307; Detroit, 1888.

https://tinyurl.com/y3r7xmaw

SCHOOLCRAFT, HENRY R., LL.D.: History, Condition and Prospects of the Indian Tribes of the United States, 5 vols., 8vo. ; Philadelphia, 1853.

https://tinyurl.com/yxs4tzk2

SEARLE, W. S., A.M., M.D.: A new form of nervous disease; together with an essay on Erythroxylon Coca, 12mo.; New York, 1881.

https://tinyurl.com/yxr55wyv

SQUIRE, E. GEORGE, M.A., F.S.A.: Peru, Incidents of Travel and Exploration in the Land of the Incas, 111., 8vo.; New York, 1877.

https://tinyurl.com/y24wnf8h

STEVENSON. W. B. : Historical and Descriptive Narrative of Twenty Years' Residence in South America, 3 vols., 8vo.; London, 1825.

https://tinyurl.com/y5qrdxo6

STEWART. F. E.: Coca leaf cigars and cigarettes; Philadelphia Medical Times, XV; 933-935; Philadelphia, 1884-85.

https://tinyurl.com/y4h27lnr

STIMMEL, A. F.: Coca in the opium and alcohol habits; Therapeutic Gazette; (n. s.), II; Detroit, 1881.

https://tinyurl.com/y3jarwwa

STOCKMAN, RALPH, M.D., F.R.C.P. : The Action of Benzoyl-ecgonine ; Journal of Anatomy and Physiology ; XXI; 46; London, 1886.

https://tinyurl.com/y6556348

SUTCLIFFE, THOMAS: Sixteen Years in Chile and Peru; London, 1841.

https://tinyurl.com/yynarnb6

TEMPLE, EDMUND: Travels in Various Parts of Peru, 2 vols.; London, 1830.

https://tinyurl.com/yyksgadd

TSCHUDI, JOHANN JACOB VON: Die Kechua Sprache, 3 pts. in 2 vols., 8vo.; Vienna, 1853.

https://tinyurl.com/y3hurtxr

TUKE, D. HACK, M.D., F.R.C.P., LL.D.: The Influence of the Mind upon the Body in Health and Disease, 2 ed., 8vo.; Philadelphia, 1884.

https://tinyurl.com/y57hot4f

UNANUE, HIPOLITO: Disertacion sobre el aspecto, cultivo, commercio y virtudes de la famosa planta del Peru nombrada Coca; Mercurio Peruano; XI, pp. 205-250; Lima, 1794.

https://tinyurl.com/y6jrxwrm

VELASCO, JUAN DE: Historia del Reino de Quito; Ternaux Cornpans; Paris, 1840.

https://tinyurl.com/y4b8b4kb

WAITZ, T.: Anthropologie der Naturvölker, III; 6 vols. ; Leipzig.

https://tinyurl.com/yym3bvcl

WHYMPER, EDWARD: Travels in the Great Andes of the Equator; New York, 1892.

**https://tinyurl.com/yxhyqv6k**

ZWAARDEMAKER, H. : Cocain-anosmie ; Fortschritte der Medicin, July 1, Berlin, 1889.

**https://tinyurl.com/y3mgryo8**

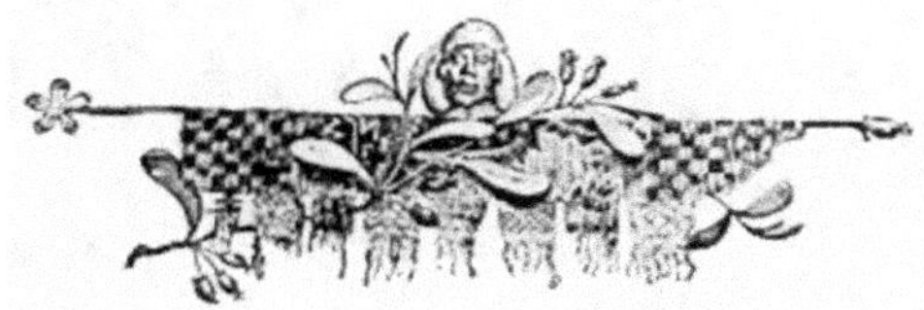

9 781699 514313